Crohn's Disease and Ulcerative Colitis

Ramona Rajapakse

Crohn's Disease and Ulcerative Colitis

A Complete Guide for Patients

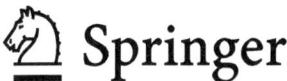 Springer

Ramona Rajapakse, MD
Mather Gastroenterology
Zucker School of Medicine at Hofstra/Northwell
Port Jefferson, NY, USA

ISBN 978-3-031-45406-6   ISBN 978-3-031-45407-3   (eBook)
https://doi.org/10.1007/978-3-031-45407-3

Illustrations by Sapphire Perera

This Springer imprint is published by the registered company Springer Nature Switzerland AG
The registered company address is: Gewerbestrasse 11, 6330 Cham, Switzerland

Paper in this product is recyclable.

Preface

During my 20 plus years as a practicing gastroenterologist specialized in inflammatory bowel disease (IBD), I get asked many questions by patients ranging from "what is Crohn's" to "what can I eat." In addition to lengthy discussions, I often draw pictures to help patients understand gastrointestinal anatomy.

For the longest time, I wanted to put down these conversations and drawings on paper, and I finally accomplished it with this book. I am delighted that you are reading this book, and I hope that you will find it informative and useful as you, or a friend/family member, negotiate living with IBD.

A special thank you to Sapphire Perera, who took my preliminary line drawings and created very special illustrations for this book.

Thanks also to Royce Perera for taking the time to read through my manuscript and make useful suggestions.

Port Jefferson, NY, USA   Ramona Rajapakse

Contents

Chapter 1
The Digestive System: Structure and Function

The digestive system is an important part of the human body because it is responsible for the breakdown, processing, and absorption of the nutrients required for proper functioning of the human body. It is also important in excreting products of digestion. The digestive system consists of the gastrointestinal (GI) tract as well as the pancreas, liver, gall bladder, and biliary system.

Structure

The GI tract consists of hollow organs that extend continuously from the mouth down to the anus. It includes the mouth, esophagus, stomach, small intestine, large intestine (also called the colon), and anus. The pancreas and liver are solid organs that produce secretions that are important for the process of digestion. The biliary system is a conduit through which bile is secreted into the gastrointestinal tract or gut. Bile is stored in the gallbladder and released when needed to aid digestion.

The small intestine is approximately 20 feet long, folded up in the abdominal cavity, and divided into three sections: The first part is called the duodenum; the second part is called the jejunum, and the third part is called the ileum. The ileum connects directly through the ileocecal valve, which is like a gate, into the first part of the colon which is called the cecum (Fig. 1.1).

The large intestine or colon is approximately 5 feet long and divided into the cecum, ascending colon, transverse colon, descending colon, sigmoid colon, and rectum. Each part of the colon is structurally slightly different and therefore prone to slightly different problems and complications. The appendix is attached to the cecum and has very little function which is why it can be removed when it gets inflamed without causing any problems.

The wall of the GI tract consists of an inner lining called the mucosa, and several other layers with a surrounding muscular layer and an outer layer called the serosa.

© The Author(s), under exclusive license to Springer Nature Switzerland AG 2023
R. Rajapakse, *Crohn's Disease and Ulcerative Colitis*,
https://doi.org/10.1007/978-3-031-45407-3_1

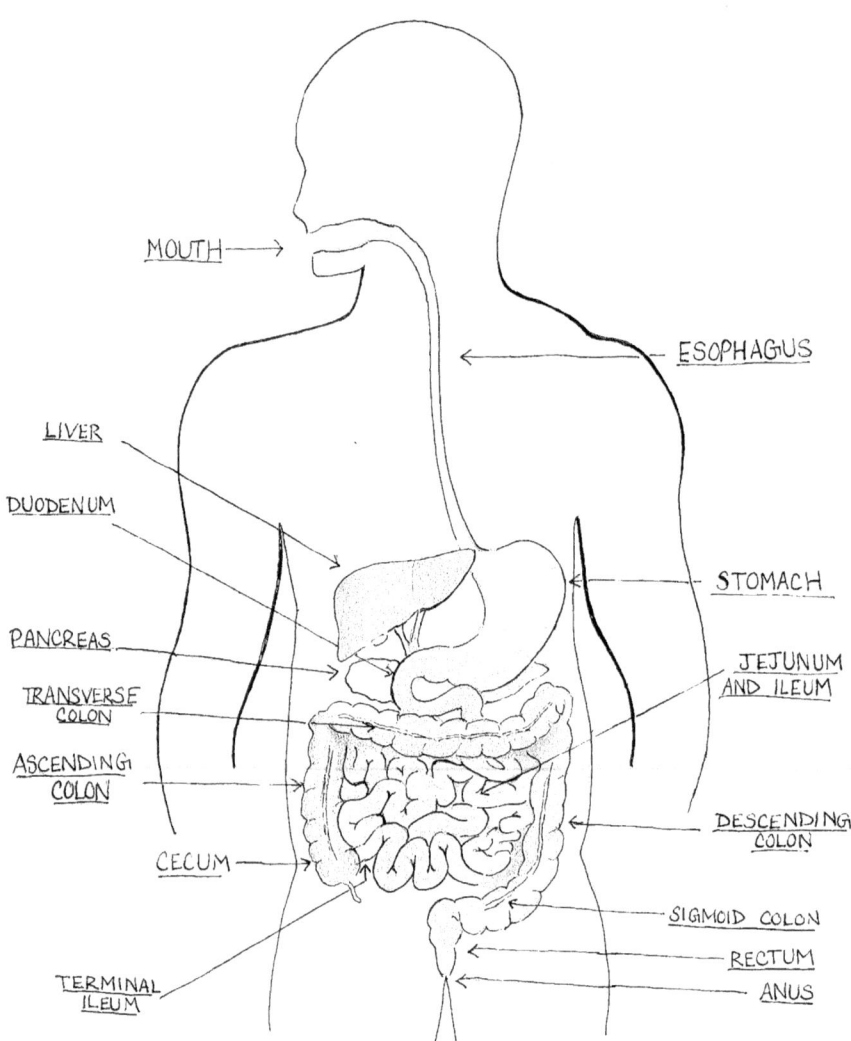

Fig. 1.1 Anatomy of the digestive tract

The mucosal layer has a variety of functions including secretion of digestive juices and hormones, and absorption of nutrients and water. The mucosal layer in the small intestine is lined with tubular structures called villi which greatly increase the surface area for absorption of nutrients. The lining of the colon, on the other hand, is relatively flat and more conducive to absorption of water (Fig. 1.2).

The small intestine and colon are filled with bacteria, which, in its entirety, is called the gut microbiome. The gut microbiome is a vital part of the human body and plays an important role in keeping the gut and the entire body in a state of health.

Fig. 1.2 Structure of the small intestine

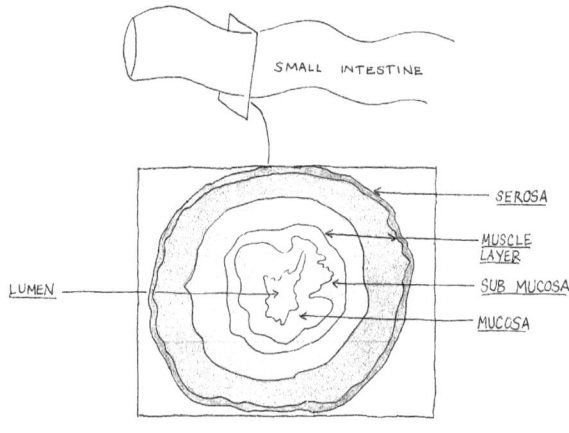

The liver is a large organ, located in the upper right abdomen, tucked under the ribs. Its main function is detoxification. It also produces substances that are important for digestion like bile. The pancreas is nestled in the middle of the abdomen. It is a slender long organ with a head, body, and tail, and a central duct that carries secretions (Fig. 1.1).

Function

Each portion of the digestive system plays an important role in digestion, absorption, and excretion. The digestive system breaks down nutrients into smaller and smaller portions which can then be absorbed through the wall of the intestine into the blood stream and distributed to all parts of the body to provide energy for cell activities. Residual substances that are not digested, and waste products of digestion are excreted finally through the large intestine into the colon and eliminated via the anus.

The mouth begins the process of digestion. Food is chewed, and saliva, produced by the salivary glands, helps to lubricate the bolus of food. The presence of taste buds in the tongue stimulates the release of various secretions that are important for digestion. The tongue helps with mixing, as well as in propulsion and swallowing of the bolus of food. The epiglottis, which is the small flap of tissue at the back of the mouth, automatically folds over the windpipe during swallowing to prevent food from entering the windpipe and causing choking.

The esophagus is mainly a conduit for passage of food from the mouth to the stomach, facilitated by a process of muscular contractions called peristalsis. This process is controlled by the nervous system and is involuntary.

When food reaches the lower esophagus, it passes through a thick layer of muscle called the lower esophageal sphincter which relaxes in order to allow food to pass into the stomach. This sphincter usually stays closed to prevent regurgitation of food and liquid from the stomach back up into the esophagus. It does relax intermittently to allow gas to escape during burping. The stomach is a relatively sterile portion of the intestine. Stomach cells produce acid which inhibits the growth of most bacteria and is also important in breaking down some nutrients. The stomach also helps to mechanically break down the food further and delivers this food to the small bowel in small quantities.

The major job of nutrient absorption occurs in the small intestine. Nutrients move along the small intestine through a process of peristalsis due to contractions and relaxation of the muscle layers. This produces not only the forward movement of nutrients, but it also allows mixing, and enhances absorption.

Bile, secreted by the liver, and enzymes and bicarbonate secreted by the pancreas, help with digestion in the small intestine. Bile is transported via bile ducts and stored in the gall bladder until it is required.

Secretions are controlled through hormones that are released locally and through control from the central and peripheral nervous systems when there is food in the intestine. Digestions and absorption are under the control of an intricate and complex neuro/hormonal system.

During digestion, proteins, fats, carbohydrates, vitamins, and minerals are broken down mechanically into small particles and then, via chemical reactions, into exceedingly small particles. These tiny particles can pass through the intestinal wall in a process called absorption. Chemical digestion occurs through the action of various enzymes produced by the pancreas and the lining of the small intestine. Proteins are broken down into amino acids and fats into fatty acids and glycerol, and carbohydrates are broken down into their simplest forms including glucose. These smaller particles of nutrients are then easily absorbed through the lining of the intestine into the blood stream from where they are carried to the liver. The liver then stores, processes, and delivers the nutrients to the rest of the body.

There is also a lymph system which forms a network around the GI tract. The lymphatics help in absorption of fats, and lymph nodes around the gut are like sentinels. They have a role in fighting infection introduced into the gut through food.

The body utilizes sugars, fats, and amino acids to produce energy for activities and also to grow, multiply, and repair cells all over the body.

When the digested food moves into the large intestine, most of the nutrients have already been absorbed. Non-digestible materials like fiber remain in the colon, together with significant amounts of fluid and bacteria. The colonic wall absorbs most of this water allowing the contents to solidify and become a formed stool. Stool is composed mostly of non-absorbable fiber, older cells from the lining of the GI tract and bacterial cell walls. This is moved along the colon through peristaltic contractions and finally evacuated from the rectum when feasible. The anus helps to control evacuation of flatus and feces at a convenient time and is usually under both voluntary and involuntary control.

In summary, the GI tract is a finely coordinated and constructed organ system that can break down nutrients, propel them, absorb and process them, store, distribute, and detoxify. It is also a first line of defense against orally ingested invading organisms.

Problems Can Occur in any Part of This Process from a Variety of Diseases, Including Crohn's Disease

Mouth: Saliva production can be decreased in Sjogren's syndrome and some other autoimmune conditions, and Crohn's can cause ulcers and inflammation.

Esophagus: GERD (gastroesophageal reflux disease) occurs when the lower esophageal sphincter becomes loose and acid contents in the stomach move up into the esophagus causing burning, pain, and regurgitation. Esophagitis, inflammation of the esophagus, can occur from GERD. Esophageal cancer, motility disorders as well as Crohn's can all affect the esophagus.

Stomach: Can be affected by inflammation (gastritis), ulcers, infections (Helicobacter Pylori), motility problems (gastroparesis), Crohn's, and cancer. This may manifest with abdominal pain, nausea, or vomiting, sometimes bleeding.

Small intestines: Crohn's, Celiac disease (inability to digest gluten), infections, cancer, and other inflammatory disorders can affect the small intestine causing problems with digestion and absorption of nutrients.

Colon: Crohn's, ulcerative colitis, cancer, ulcers, other inflammatory conditions can cause diarrhea and bleeding.

Liver, biliary tract, and gall bladder: Hepatitis (infections, inflammation), bile duct problems, gall stones, cirrhosis, Crohn's, and ulcerative colitis (extra intestinal manifestation).

Pancreas: Inflammation of the pancreas, called pancreatitis, can occur due to a variety of causes. Pancreatic cancer is a serious condition. Crohn's can occasionally affect the pancreas, it is more common for some of the medications used to treat Crohn's to cause pancreatic inflammation and should always be considered if there is abdominal pain.

Chapter 2
Crohn's Disease and Ulcerative Colitis: Definitions and Symptoms

Crohn's disease (CD) and ulcerative colitis (UC) are chronic inflammatory diseases of the GI tract and are together termed inflammatory bowel disease (IBD). There are several differences between the two, but about 10–20% of patients do not fit neatly into either category and are considered to have indeterminate colitis.

IBD affects 1.6–3 million Americans, and the incidence appears to be increasing globally. There also appears to be a rising incidence of CD in the pediatric population, of uncertain cause.

IBD can present for the first time at any age. However, the peak age for CD is in the second decade of life and for UC in the third decade. In pediatric patients, CD appears to be more common while the elderly seems to suffer more with UC. IBD affects both sexes equally. Although there is a predilection for Ashkenazi Jews, incidence of iBD is rising in other ethnic groups, especially with migration and globalization.

In general, although there are exceptions, patients who are diagnosed at a younger age seem to have a more aggressive course than those who are diagnosed later in life. Early intervention and appropriate therapy are therefore very important in order to prevent complications.

IBD is a chronic condition with periods of relapse and remission. Although it can have a significant effect on the quality of life, it doesn't usually result in early death. The clinical symptoms depend on the type of IBD, location of inflammation, and the presence or absence of manifestations outside the GI tract. There is often a delay in diagnosis with patients, especially the young, being carried with a diagnosis of irritable bowel syndrome (predominantly a problem with motility of the gut rather than inflammation) for many months and sometimes years.

R. Rajapakse, *Crohn's Disease and Ulcerative Colitis*, https://doi.org/10.1007/978-3-031-45407-3_2

Crohn's Disease (CD)

Crohn's disease was first described by Dr. Crohn, together with his colleagues Dr. Ginsberg and Dr. Oppenheimer, in 1932.

Crohn's disease can affect any part of the GI tract, from the mouth down to the anus, but most commonly affects the ileum (*ileitis*), the ileum and colon(*ileocolitis*), jejunum and ileum (*jejunoileitis*), or the colon alone(colitis). It tends to affect the stomach and the upper part of the small bowel in young people (*gastroduodenitis*). Typically, the inflammation tends to be patchy with normal intervening areas of mucosa. These patches of inflammation are called *skip lesions*. Inflammation produces ulcers in the mucosa, with surrounding swelling and redness. Tiny ulcers are called "aphthous" ulcers. There may be a tendency to bleed from these ulcers, sometimes only in microscopic amounts (Fig. 2.1).

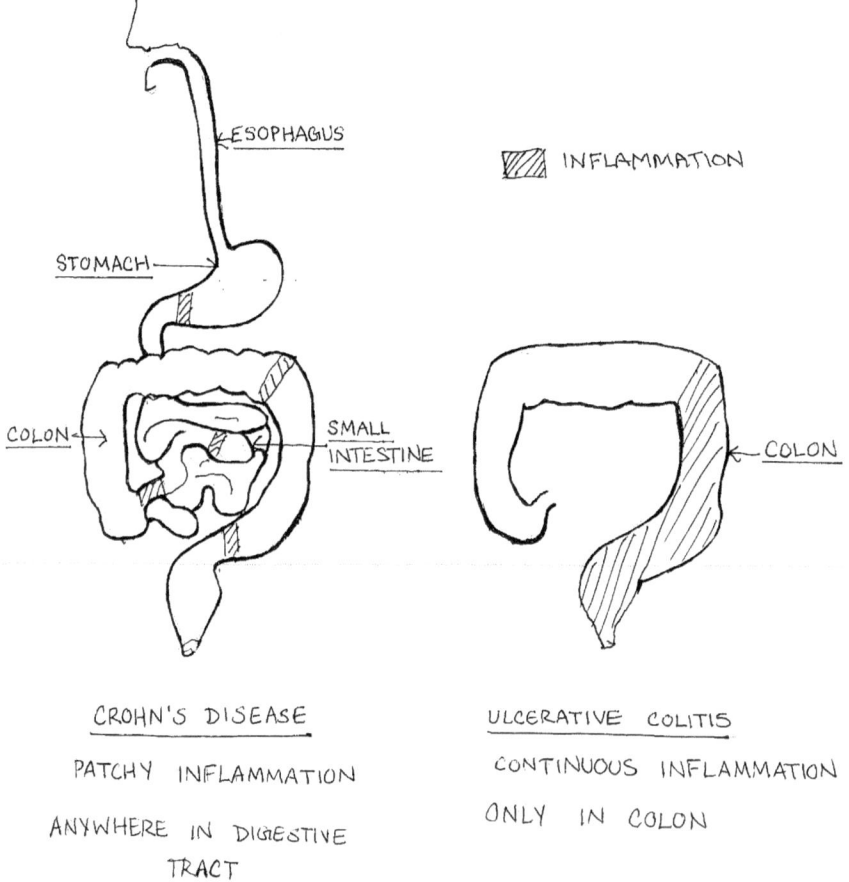

Fig. 2.1 Differences between Crohn's and colitis

Inflammation usually starts in the innermost lining of the gut and extends through the wall of the gut producing complications. If the inflammation extends through the wall of the gut, it can produce communication with adjoining bowel, urinary bladder, vagina, or skin, through *fistulas*. This is discussed elsewhere. Chronic inflammation of the bowel wall can result in narrowing and scar tissue producing stenosis or stricture. Crohn's disease may produce anal and rectal complications.

Crohn's is also associated with manifestations outside the gut, called extra intestinal manifestations, as detailed in another chapter.

Symptoms

These vary depending on the site and severity of inflammation and can be mild or severe. Sometimes there can be inflammation brewing for months or years with little in the way of symptoms. Symptoms can come on gradually or appear all of a sudden. Symptoms may be continuous or sporadic and intermittent. There may or may not be an association of symptoms with food intake. Symptoms also depend on the presence or absence of complications.

Ileocolitis

This is the most common site for inflammation and affects the terminal ileum and any part of the colon. Symptoms can include abdominal pain, abdominal cramping, and diarrhea which may or may not be bloody. The pain may be mid abdominal or localized to the lower right part of the abdomen. There may be low grade fevers, loss of appetite and therefore significant weight loss.

Ileitis

In this case, the inflammation is localized to the last part of the small intestine, the ileum. Symptoms are similar to those outlined above. In severe cases, if the inflammation extends through the wall of the intestine, there may be an inflammatory mass or pus pocket located in that area producing pain and fevers. Fistulas may also form.

Gastroduodenal Crohn's

In this case, inflammation affects the stomach and first part of the small intestine, the duodenum. Symptoms are predominantly upper abdominal pain and discomfort, nausea, vomiting, loss of appetite, and weight loss.

Jejunoileitis

This is Crohn's inflammation of the mid small bowel. Abdominal pain is the main symptom which can be crampy and particularly intense after meals. Again, diarrhea with or without blood may be a feature and fistulas and abscesses may form. Narrowing may occur causing nausea, vomiting, and abdominal pain.

Crohn's Colitis

In this case, inflammation occurs only in the colon. The predominant symptom is diarrhea, sometimes with pain and bleeding.

Perianal Crohn's

In this condition, there are skin tags, hemorrhoids, ulcers, fissures, and/or fistulas around the anus. Skin tags are small bumps around the anus that can become larger during a flare. Hemorrhoids are enlarged blood vessels that can bleed sometimes and also occur very commonly in the general population. A fissure is a tear and can be very painful. Fistulas around the anus typically originate from the rectum and can leak stool and mucus. There may also be painful pockets of pus, called perianal abscesses around the anus.

Crohn's inflammation does not have to remain in one part of the body but can spread if not adequately treated.

Other symptoms can be related to nutritional deficiencies due to decreased absorption, such as anemia, as well as mineral and vitamin deficiencies, particularly Vitamin B12 deficiency. Anemia may occur due to inability to absorb iron or loss of iron through bleeding. Anemia can also occur if vitamin B12 absorption is impaired due to inflammation in the terminal ileum. Potassium and magnesium deficiency can lead to muscle weakness, while zinc deficiency can cause loss of smell and skin lesions. Vitamin B12 deficiency can lead to anemia and neurological symptoms. Vitamin A is important for the proper functioning of the eye. Vitamin D is important for bones, and vitamin K is important for blood coagulation.

Severe ileitis can predispose to kidney stones, particularly calcium oxalate stones. This presents with pain in the region of the kidneys, in the lower back with urgent desire to urinate and blood in the urine.

Ulcerative Colitis (UC)

This is a chronic inflammatory condition that affects only the colon within the GI tract. Other parts of the GI tract are not typically affected but there may be extra intestinal features.

It also differs from CD in that inflammation only affects the inner most lining layer (the mucosa) and is continuous, without skip lesions. The inflammation does not spread through the bowel wall, and therefore there are no fistulas or narrowings produced. The severity of symptoms depends on the extent and severity of inflammation.

Patients typically present with abdominal cramping and diarrhea which is more commonly bloody compared to CD. There may also be loss of appetite and weight loss.

UC is described based on the location of inflammation within the colon:

Proctitis: This is inflammation of only the rectum. Symptoms can include urgency of stool (when you have to go you have to run) and a sense of incomplete evacuation of the bowels (never feels like the bowel movement is complete). Sometimes constipation rather than diarrhea is predominant. There may also be passage of mucus and blood alone.

Left sided colitis: Affects the rectum, sigmoid, descending colon, and sometimes a little part of the transverse colon. Diarrhea is a predominant feature with or without bleeding and pain.

Pancolitis: This is where the entire colon is inflamed. Again, diarrhea and cramping with or without blood are the predominant feature (Fig. 2.1 and Tables 2.1 and 2.2).

Hemorrhoids

These can occur in both UC and CD. These are swollen veins in the lower part of the anus. Sometimes they protrude only during a bowel movement and go back in afterwards. Sometimes they remain out all the time.

Causes of Hemorrhoids

Straining during bowel movements.
Straining while lifting something heavy.

Table 2.1 Main differences between UC and Crohn's in terms of disease activity

Ulcerative colitis	Crohn's disease
Only affects the colon	Can affect any part of the GI tract
Only affects the inner lining (mucosa)	Can affect the whole wall (transmural)
No fistulas	Can cause fistulas
No abscesses (pus pockets)	Can cause abscesses
No strictures (narrowing)	Can cause strictures
Manifestations outside the GI tract	Manifestations outside the GI tract
"Cured" with surgery	No cure with surgery

Table 2.2 Main differences in potential symptoms between Crohn's and UC

Crohn's disease	Ulcerative colitis
Less prominent diarrhea/bleeding	Bloody diarrhea and mucus common
Abdominal pain is prominent	Less abdominal pain
Nausea and vomiting	Less likely to have nausea and vomiting
Chronic fever and weight loss	Less prominent weight loss and fever
Anorectal pain and discharge	Usually, no anal pain or discharge

Pregnancy (the weight of the uterus presses on the veins).
Anal sex.
Severe constipation/diarrhea.

Symptoms of Hemorrhoids

Bulging and anal itching are common symptoms. Sometimes they cause bleeding. If the blood inside a hemorrhoid clots, producing a thrombosed hemorrhoid, it becomes very painful. Hemorrhoids can go away on their own but if they are bothersome, they may need treatment.

Treatments for Hemorrhoids

1. Maintain regular bowel habit by eating fruits and vegetables, using fiber supplements and drinking plenty of water (64 oz. (about 1.89 L) per day).
2. Exercise regularly as this aids bowel movements.
3. Preparation H ointment and suppositories, available over the counter, can help to shrink the hemorrhoids.
4. Prescription strength medication with a steroid (Anusol HC) can be prescribed by a physician to shrink hemorrhoids.
5. If medication and lifestyle measures do not resolve the hemorrhoids, or if there is significant bleeding and pain, referral to a colorectal surgeon may be necessary for further treatment.

Complications of Crohn's Disease and Ulcerative Colitis

Intestinal Obstruction

If a Crohn's stricture becomes severe, it can produce a partial or complete bowel obstruction. This can cause severe abdominal swelling, pain, nausea, and vomiting together with decreased passage of gas and stool. Although obstruction may resolve with conservative measures such as avoiding food, if it persists, it may require surgery to remove the narrowed segment of intestine. Sometimes the stricture is chronic, does not produce a complete obstruction, and can be managed with dietary modification such as avoidance of high fiber foods (a low fiber diet) (see Appendix).

Fistulas

These occur only in CD and not in UC and consist of an abnormal connection between one part of the intestine and another, or with another organ. The most common fistulas are located in the anal region. If there is an enteroenteric fistula, nutrients may bypass areas for absorption resulting in malnutrition. Fistulas may only be diagnosed with a CT scan or MRI. If there is a fistula into the bladder, it can cause passage of air and stool with urine and recurrent urinary tract infections (Fig. 2.2). If there is a fistula into the vagina, it can cause air and stool passage through the vagina. A fistula into the skin will cause a visible opening in the skin with leakage of stool.

Fistulas can become infected and produce pockets of pus called abscesses which can be painful and life threatening. If an abscess occurs, it should be drained and treated with antibiotics.

Perianal Disease

In Crohn's disease, in addition to anal fistulas, one can get large skin tags and anal fissures. The fissures are minute cracks around the anal opening and can be painful and bleed. The skin tags can become irritated. Abscesses can cause life threatening infection.

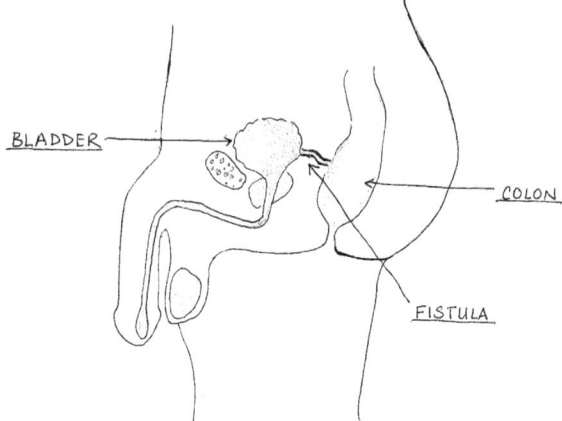

Fig. 2.2 Fistula from colon to bladder (colovesical fistula)

Malnutrition

Diarrhea and abdominal cramping can cause a loss of appetite leading to malnutrition. In addition, inflammation of areas of the intestine that are important for nutrient absorption can also lead to malabsorption of nutrients. Ileitis can lead to an inability to absorb vitamin B12. Inability to absorb some other vitamins can contribute to bone loss especially in long standing disease.

Anemia

In both Crohn's disease and UC, anemia can develop due to loss of blood or inability to absorb iron and B12.

Cancer

CD of the small intestine can be associated with an increased risk of lymphoma and small bowel cancer. If there is perianal disease, there is also an increased risk of cancer around the anus. If there is colonic involvement, there is an increased risk of colon cancer.

UC is associated with an increased risk of colon cancer.

Manifestations Outside the GI Tract (Extra Intestinal Manifestations)

IBD can be associated with inflammation in other parts of the body including the eyes, skin, liver, and joints. This is discussed at length in Chap. 13.

Complications Related to Treatment of IBD

This will be discussed at length in other chapters but can include low white cell counts, infections, allergic type reactions, and increased risk of cancer.

Chapter 3
Cause(s) of Crohn's and Ulcerative Colitis: Genetic and Environmental Influences

We have come a long way in our understanding of IBD, but we still don't know exactly why some people develop IBD and others don't.

What we do know is that the cause is multifactorial: a combination of genetic, immunological, and environmental factors.

Figure 3.1 (Interplay of genetic, environmental factors).

Genetic Factors

Over the past couple of decades, our understanding of the genetic influences on IBD has increased greatly, in large part from studies within ethnic and family groups. In CD, 2–14% and in UC 7–11% of patients report having a family member with the same disease.

If there is a first degree relative with IBD (mother, father, brother, sister), there is a tenfold increased risk of developing IBD compared with families without IBD. If both parents have IBD, the risk to the child is approximately 30%.

Genome wide association studies (GWAS) have helped to identify some of the genes associated with IBD. GWAS is a process where scientists can study the DNA of a large group of people in order to determine small variations called single nucleotide polymorphisms (SNPs). Using this technique, more than 200 genes associated with IBD have been identified and more are being found on an ongoing basis. Most of these genes play a role in the barrier function of the intestine and how the intestine reacts to bacteria and viruses.

NOD2 was the first gene identified for CD and is located on chromosome 16. However, its exact role has yet to be determined. Interestingly, it is not implicated in UC. There are more than 100 genes identified with an association with UC. We don't routinely check for any of these genes because the presence of the gene does not mean that one will develop IBD, and the absence of the gene does not mean that

R. Rajapakse, *Crohn's Disease and Ulcerative Colitis*,
https://doi.org/10.1007/978-3-031-45407-3_3

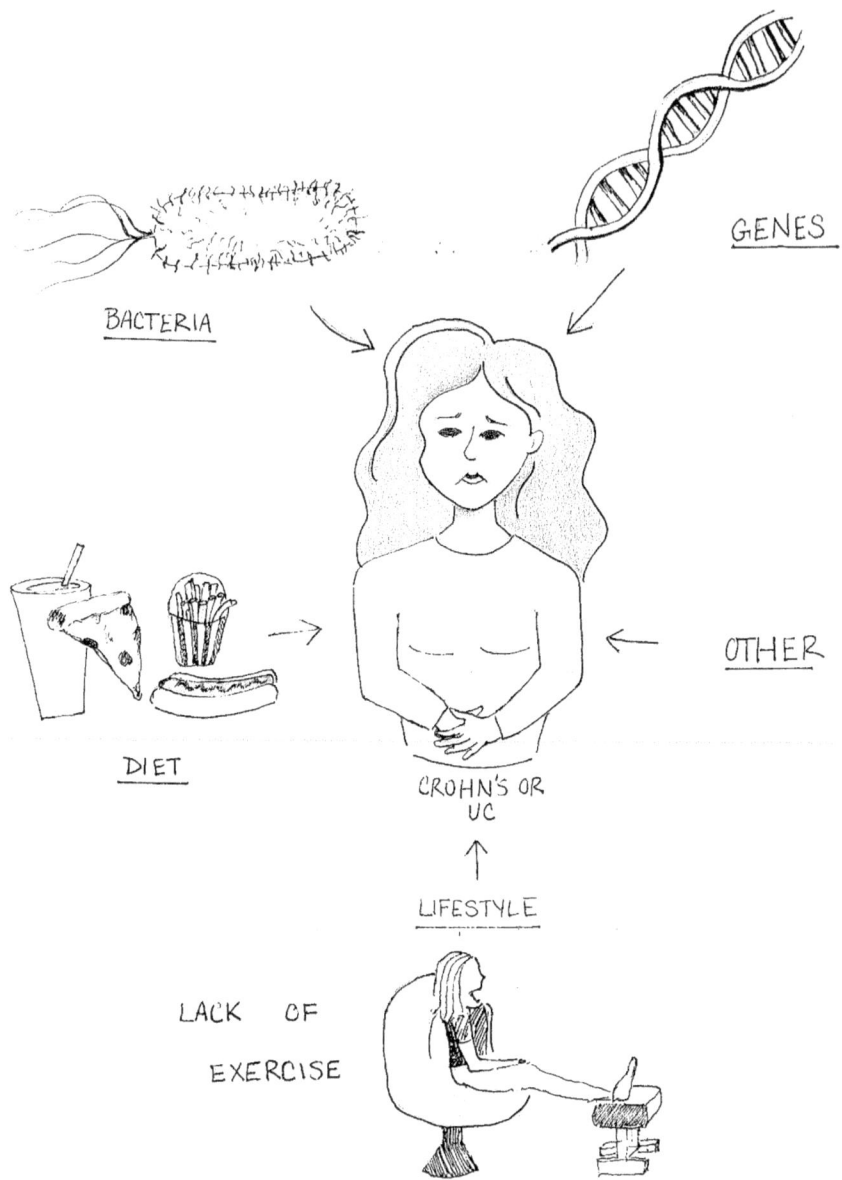

Fig. 3.1 Cause of IBD—multifactorial

one will never get IBD. This is because there are multiple factors at play in the pathogenesis of IBD.

Lifestyle

Smoking

Cigarette smoking is associated with an increased risk of CD, and with worsening disease in those who already have CD. On the other hand, it is associated with a decreased risk of UC and sometimes patients present for the first time with UC after smoking cessation. There are likely to be other factors associated with this, including genetic and ethnic factors. The exact mechanism for this is unknown but smoking can cause changes in immune responses and also affects the gut microbiome, and this may play a role in how it makes particularly Crohn's worse because gut microbiome variations are more pronounced in CD.

Diet

There is evidence that a high fiber diet is protective for Crohn's disease while a diet high in red meat is associated with an increased risk of UC. It may be that the hemoglobin in red meat can damage the intestinal epithelium. There is also evidence that a western diet that is high in processed foods, processed grains, animal and red protein and low in fruits and vegetables is associated with an increased risk of IBD. Cultures with a high consumption of fiber typically have a lower incidence of IBD although these differences are becoming less marked with migration, travel, and westernization of diet.

Green tea may have some anti-inflammatory properties in the gut. In addition to direct actions on the epithelium, diet can affect the microbes in the gut, and this may play a role in changing the risk for IBD.

Several dietary interventions have been popularized in the past several years. Although these diets can reduce symptoms of IBD, they do not clearly reduce inflammation. In the pediatric CD population, however, the use of elemental diets has been shown to reduce inflammation. An elemental diet is a liquid in which nutrition is broken down to its elements. Unfortunately, it is not very well tolerated for long-term use.

The Microbiome

The gut microbiome consists of all the microorganisms that live within the GI tract including bacteria, fungi, and viruses. The microbiome starts to be formed after birth and, like a fingerprint, is unique to the individual. As our understanding of the gut microbiome has grown, we have realized that it is very important for our overall health and can affect many different body systems, not just the gut. These microbes in the gut help with digestion, produce useful agents, and protect against intestinal pathogens. They protect against gut pathogens by inducing the immune cells in the gut. They also help to prevent the immune system from overacting to other microbes. In addition, they help to maintain the integrity of the lining of the intestine. The relationship between the microbes themselves and between the microbiome and the host is complex.

In patients with IBD, there appears to be a change in the microbiome with a decrease in diversity of organisms. There are more pro-inflammatory microbes and less anti-inflammatory microbes. These differences seem to be most pronounced with Crohn's. Patients with UC have a more normal microbiome. Similarly, there are changes in the composition of fungi and viruses as well. There appears to be a higher population of candida (yeast) in patients with IBD and this is reflected in some of the blood tests that are used for diagnosis. However, this finding does not have a practical implication for treatment. What we don't know is whether the microbiome becomes altered because of inflammation or whether the inflammation is caused by an altered microbiome. Further studies are needed to clarify this.

Probiotics are live organisms that are available over the counter and have beneficial properties when ingested orally. They are helpful in irritable bowel syndrome and may have some benefit in IBD as well by improving the microbiome.

Stress and Mental Health

It is well known that stress can have an effect on bowel habits. This is well recognized in irritable bowel syndrome (IBS), but it also plays a role in IBD. Under stressful situations, many people experience diarrhea. It is now known that stress can actually affect the lining of the intestine and produce low grade inflammation and irritation through release of inflammatory chemicals. The gut–brain axis consists of neuronal connections between the gut and the brain. The nerve cells can induce the release of chemicals within the gut wall resulting in inflammation. There is a higher rate of depression in patients with IBD compared to the general population. This is likely a response to having a chronic illness, but it can prolong and prevent healing. Use of anti-depressant medications can help to improve IBD not only through improving the mental outlook of the patient but also through modulation of gut chemicals and reducing the perception of pain.

Low Vitamin D

Lack of Vitamin D causes bone loss. In addition, it has been implicated in a variety of illnesses including cardiovascular disease, cognitive impairment, and IBD. Vitamin D plays a role in the immune system. There have been studies that show a lack of vitamin D resulting in more pronounced IBD disease activity, but a causative association has not been made. Vitamin D deficiency can result from poor absorption from the gut, decreased intake (especially of dairy such as in patients with lactose intolerance or those on un-supplemented vegan diets), and reduced sun exposure.

Non-steroidal Anti-inflammatory Agents (NSAIDs)

NSAIDs are a group of medications that reduce some types of inflammation and are therefore used for the treatment of pain (especially when there is an inflammatory component) and arthritis. Most NSAIDs, such as ibuprofen (Advil) and naproxen (Aleve) are widely available over the counter. These medications are known to cause ulcers and inflammation in the stomach and small intestine, but they can also aggravate preexisting IBD, but there is no evidence that they cause IBD. NSAIDs should be avoided, if possible, by patients with IBD.

Vaccines

There have been many concerns raised about vaccines. In relation to IBD, there was concern about whether vaccination predisposes to IBD. To date there is no evidence that any vaccination leads to IBD. Therefore, all patients should have age-appropriate vaccination. Live vaccines should not be used in patients who are on immunomodulators and biologics.

There are various other factors that have been evaluated as causative agents for IBD. Thus far none has been definitively confirmed.

In summary, IBD is believed to be caused by an exaggerated immune response triggered by an unknown agent, in a genetically predisposed individual.

Chapter 4
Diagnostic Testing

Just as there is no single cause of IBD, there is no single test available that provides a definitive diagnosis of IBD. Diagnosis of IBD is made using a combination of factors including a careful history and physical examination by a gastroenterologist, radiological testing, endoscopic testing, and lab testing. The final diagnosis is made by the gastroenterologist using a composite of findings. Although sometimes the diagnosis is very clear, sometimes the diagnosis may not be clear or apparent initially and may take a while to make. Sometimes a patient appears to have UC and later manifests features of CD, and vice versa, requiring a change in diagnosis. Although a change in diagnosis does not affect medical treatment very much, it can affect surgical treatment if it is required.

Lab Testing

Lab tests include blood tests and stool tests. Blood tests will check for anemia with the hemoglobin level (CBC: complete blood count), for electrolyte problems and kidney problems from diarrhea (CMP: complete metabolic panel) and for any abnormal liver function tests (hepatic function panel). There are inflammatory markers called C reactive protein (CRP) and erythrocyte sedimentation rate (ESR), which may be elevated. Sometimes the CRP is normal even with inflammation and ESR may be elevated due to other reasons.

Stool should be checked for microorganisms, including C. difficile, as well as for blood and inflammatory markers. C. difficile is an acquired infection that may be silent for a prolonged period and suddenly become active with use of antibiotics. It can produce profuse diarrhea and abdominal pain and should be treated with antibiotics. It is a great mimicker of IBD. Stool calprotectin is a marker of inflammation in the intestine. Low levels rule out inflammation, but high levels do not necessarily mean there is inflammation unless they are very high. It is therefore useful in trying

© The Author(s), under exclusive license to Springer Nature
Switzerland AG 2023
R. Rajapakse, *Crohn's Disease and Ulcerative Colitis*,
https://doi.org/10.1007/978-3-031-45407-3_4

to differentiate IBD from IBS in patients with diarrhea. It can also be used as a non-invasive way to monitor disease activity.

There are blood tests that can help to differentiate UC from CD (in combination with other tests), but they are not useful for the primary diagnosis of IBD. These include anti-Saccharomyces antibody (ASCA) and anti-neutrophil anti-body (ANCA).

Imaging

Radiological imaging can be useful in diagnosing and determining the extent of Crohn's disease, and in diagnosing complications in both CD and UC. In times past, small bowel series and small bowel follow throughs were performed but now the most commonly used imaging modalities are CT scans and MRIs.

CT scan is a technique where a series of X-rays are beamed around the body from different angles. A computer then makes a composite of the images. If intravenous contrast is being used, an intravenous catheter is introduced into the arm for administration. Oral contrast is also usually required. The CT scan of the abdomen and pelvis looks at all the organs within the abdominal cavity. It is particularly useful for diagnosing complications of IBD such as abscesses and masses.

CT enterography is a special type of CT scan that specifically looks at the small bowel and is useful in determining small bowel activity in Crohn's disease. Technically, as far as the patient is concerned, it is similar to a regular CT scan of the abdomen, but it is performed differently, and the images obtained are specific to the small intestine. It typically requires drinking 1.5–2 L of a contrast agent which helps to distend the intestine and produce detailed images of the small intestine and wall and takes about 5–10 min.

CT scans are associated with radiation exposure and should not therefore be performed too frequently in a short space of time, especially in young patients. Sometimes patients go to multiple different emergency rooms over a short period of time. The emergency room physicians may be unaware of recent imaging and will order repeat imaging. It is important that patients are aware of the risks of too many CT scans and inform their healthcare providers if they have had recent imaging.

MRI uses radio waves rather than regular radiation and requires intravenous and oral contrast as well. It takes about 30–45 min, and it produces detailed images of the small bowel.

MR enterography also produces detailed images of the small intestine and can help to distinguish active inflammation from scar tissue. Unfortunately, it cannot be done in an open MRI so if there is a problem with claustrophobia, it cannot be done. It cannot be performed if there is metal in the body as well.

Both of these imaging modalities can diagnose strictures, fistulas, abscesses, and the presence or absence of inflammation.

Kidney injury can occasionally occur with the use of intravenous contrast, especially in people who have pre-existing kidney problems and the radiologist will do a blood test to determine this prior to the procedure.

Endoscopy

This is a minimally invasive technique used to examine the hollow parts of the digestive tract. It utilizes a long thin tube, called an endoscope, that is equipped with a camera, a light source and biopsy, and suction channel. The typical endoscopic examinations used in IBD include EGD for evaluation of the upper GI tract, colonoscopy for evaluation of the colon, and capsule endoscopy for evaluation of the small intestine. Other endoscopic procedures that may be necessary include ERCP (for evaluation of the bile ducts) and small bowel enteroscopy to evaluate the small intestine. If there is any abnormality, samples are taken via a biopsy forceps which is a small clip device that is introduced through the scope. This is called taking a biopsy. If there are polyps, they are removed using a small metal lasso which is also introduced through the scope. The specimens are then sent to the lab where a pathologist views them under a microscope and makes a report.

These procedures are typically performed under sedation with propofol, which is administered by an anesthesiologist via an intravenous cannula during the procedure. Potential major complications include medication reactions, perforation (making a hole in the bowel), and bleeding. All of these are rare and can be treated.

Upper Endoscopy (EGD)

There is no preparation involved except nothing to eat and drink after midnight. This procedure involves the introduction of the tube through the mouth, via the esophagus into the stomach and duodenum. The procedure itself is very fast and usually takes 5–10 min. These areas are studied for inflammation and ulcers, and biopsies are taken (Fig. 4.1).

Colonoscopy

The patient has to drink a laxative preparation the day before the procedure in order to clean out the colon. If this is not done properly, a "poor prep" is produced, obscuring the lining of the wall. Different colonoscopy preparations are available and are typically ingested the day before, in a split dose regimen. This produces diarrhea, sometimes with a little cramping. A good preparation is when the stool becomes clear, like urine. In the endoscopy unit, after sedation, the scope is introduced into the colon, and advanced all the way to the cecum (the end of the colon) and the terminal ileum (Fig. 4.2).

Fig. 4.1 Upper endoscopy

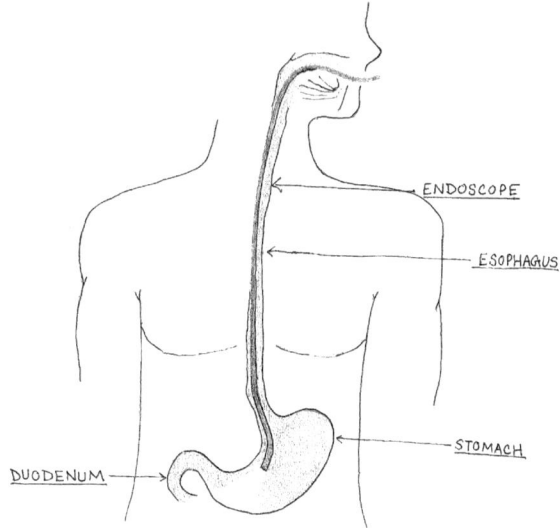

Fig. 4.2 Colonoscopy

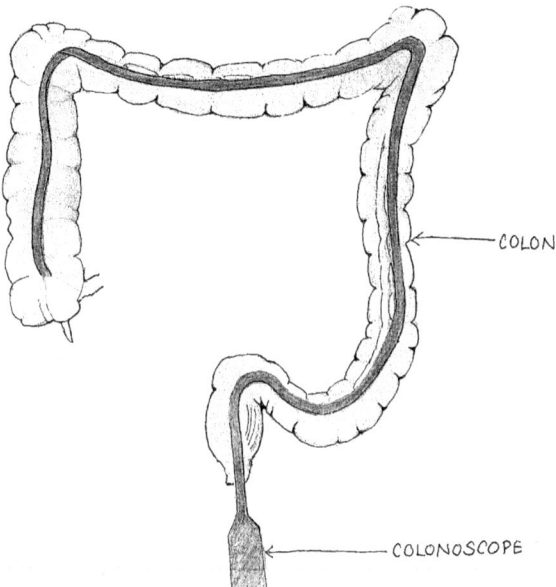

Capsule Endoscopy

This study is used to evaluate the small intestine and is usually initiated in the office. There is a small preparation to drink beforehand, but less than is required for a colonoscopy. The patient has a monitor attached, with a belt and a "handbag," and then swallows the capsule with a little water usually in the office. This is the size of a large vitamin pill (1 cm by 2 cm). The capsule has LED lights, a battery, and a transmitting device for pictures. It tumbles through the small intestine and transmits images to the monitor which is worn for 8 h. Drinking is allowed 2 h after swallowing the capsule. The monitor is taken off after 8 h and returned to the GI office the next day, and the images are downloaded onto a computer in video format. The capsule is eliminated with the stool and does not have to be retrieved. The physician can view the entire small intestine on the video imaging. The only major potential complication of this procedure is that it can get stuck if there is a narrowing in the GI tract. It is rare for this to happen to someone who has no symptoms suggestive of obstruction. If this does happen, the capsule may have to be retrieved using an endoscope or very occasionally may require surgery (Fig. 4.3 and Table 4.1).

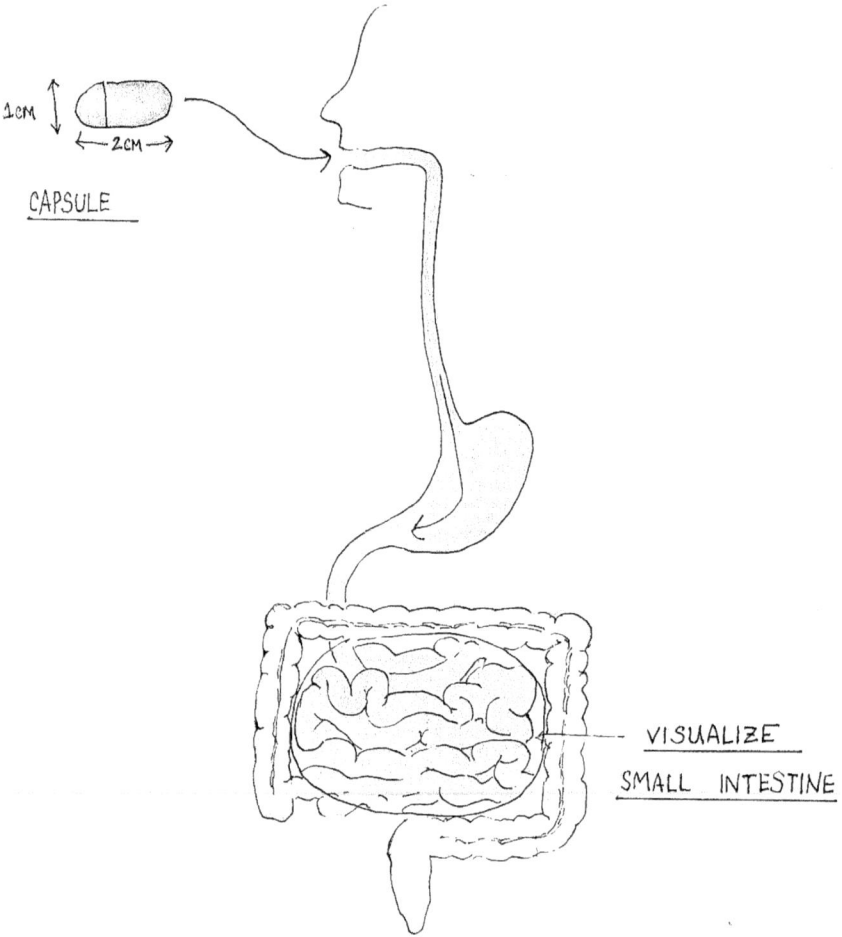

1CM

←—2CM—→

CAPSULE

VISUALIZE

SMALL INTESTINE

Fig. 4.3 Capsule endoscopy

Table 4.1 Potential tests and findings for diagnosis of IBD

Test	Findings
Stool tests	Infections, increased calprotectin
Blood tests	Anemia, increased white cell count
Upper endoscopy(EGD)	Inflammation in stomach
Colonoscopy	Patchy vs continuous inflammation in colon
Biopsies	Confirm chronic inflammation
Imaging (MRI/CT)	Show inflammation in small and large bowel
Capsule endoscopy	Small intestine inflammation

Chapter 5
Medical Treatments for Crohn's and Colitis

The mainstay of treatment for IBD is medication, which helps to control inflammation and therefore alleviate symptoms. There is no medication as yet that will cure IBD for good. All the medications available control the disease process, reduce inflammation, and bring the mucosa back to normal and therefore alleviate symptoms. However, if the medication is stopped, the inflammation will recur. This is similar to many other chronic medical conditions like asthma, diabetes, and high blood pressure which are all controlled, but not cured forever, with medication. Therefore, it is important to remain on medication. Very occasionally, however, certain patients may go into remission for a lengthy period and remain well for an extended period off medication.

IBD can cause many complications as outlined in earlier chapters, so it is important to start on the right medication early to prevent these from happening. Once complications start happening, they may be hard to reverse with medication and may require surgery.

Blood markers for inflammation such as CRP and ESR can indicate active inflammation and are useful whenever patients have symptoms. There are blood tests for markers being developed that will help to predict which patient will respond to which particular drug, but for now, the choice of medication depends on the severity and location of the disease, and on patient dependent factors.

Disease dependent factors: The type of IBD (Crohn's or ulcerative colitis), the severity, duration and extent of inflammation, presence or absence of complications, presence of manifestations outside the GI tract, and the presence of other medical conditions can dictate which medication is best.

Patient dependent factors: Age, sex, fertility and pregnancy issues and concerns, cost/insurance, and patient preference all affect choice of medication.

Since "one size does not fit all," the physician must find the right medicine for each patient. We call this *precision medicine* or *personalized medicine.*

In general, if one medication does not work, another may be added, or the patient may be switched to a different drug altogether. In the absence of adverse or allergic

© The Author(s), under exclusive license to Springer Nature Switzerland AG 2023

R. Rajapakse, *Crohn's Disease and Ulcerative Colitis*, https://doi.org/10.1007/978-3-031-45407-3_5

reactions, it is important to use each drug in an optimal manner, checking levels and increasing the dose if necessary, before discarding it for something else, because there aren't an infinite number of medications available. However, as our understanding of IBD increases, there are also numerous new and improved medications in development.

We divide up management of IBD into induction of remission and maintenance of remission. Certain drugs are used for induction, while others are used to maintain remission. Some drugs can do both.

There are two different approaches to management of inflammatory bowel disease, the *"top-down"* approach and the *"bottom up"* approach. The *top-down* approach uses advanced therapies early in the course of disease in order to prevent complications while the *bottom-up* approach uses the mildest medications first and then advances therapy as needed. There are advantages and disadvantages to both approaches. The current thinking is that management of each patient should be individualized. Patients who appeared to have more aggressive disease should start early with immunomodulators and biologics to prevent complications of disease, whereas patients with milder disease may have gradually advancing therapy to keep costs down and prevent complications of the treatment.

Currently available medical treatments:

1. 5 Amino salicylates (5-ASAs)
2. Biologics
3. Steroids
4. Immunomodulators
5. Targeted small molecules
6. Antibiotics

5-Amino Salicylates (5-ASAs)

These are orally or rectally administered medications that are primarily used for the treatment of colonic inflammation, either ulcerative colitis or Crohn's colitis. Some preparations may be used for small bowel or ileal disease, but the data for effectiveness in this situation is limited. They are used for milder disease and are generally the first line of therapy. The oral tablets are mostly coated to protect the drug from stomach acid and intestinal digestion and release their active components in the colon. It is not uncommon for entire tablets to be evacuated in the stool but, to be effective, at least 50% of the tablets should be retained.

The rectal preparations are in the form of enemas or suppositories and are used to treat inflammation in the lowest part of the colon, the left colon, sigmoid, and rectum. These rectal formulations are like a "cream" for the colon; they coat the mucosa, thus helping to reduce inflammation. When an enema is inserted, it is important to lay on your left side for at least 15 min to allow the medication to adequately coat the colon. If it comes out, a second enema can be inserted.

These medications can take a few weeks to take full effect and are generally well tolerated. They can occasionally worsen diarrhea, so it is important to bring to the attention of your doctor if the diarrhea worsens after starting the medication. Although they are considered mild drugs, 5-ASAs can have many potentially serious, albeit rare, side effects including kidney and liver disease, inflammation of the lungs and heart, and hair loss. Your doctor will inquire about possible side effects while you are on these medications and will also draw regular lab work to check for kidney and liver problems.

The oldest drug in this category is *sulfasalazine*. It contains sulfur and is therefore contraindicated in patients with sulfur allergies. In addition to the side effects listed above, when sulfasalazine is taken by men, it can cause changes in sperm, therefore reducing fertility. This is reversible within a couple of months of stopping the drug. It is therefore important to inform your doctor If you are a couple trying to get pregnant.

There are many newer formulations of 5-ASAs including generic mesalamine, *Asacol*, *Colazal*, *Lialda*, *Apriso*, and *Pentasa*. They may have to be taken several times a day or once a day depending on the drug formulation and its coating. The active drug is released in the colon except Asacol(released in the ileum) and Pentasa (released in the stomach). Asacol and Pentasa may be prescribed for small intestinal disease although they are not as effective as other medications in this location.

5-ASAs can take a few weeks to take full effect so they can only be used as first-line treatment for mild disease or as a maintenance treatment.

Biologics

This is a class of drugs that are produced from living systems such as animal cells, plant cells, or microorganisms. They are proteins and are designed to work on certain parts of the immune system. Because they are proteins, they can easily be destroyed by extremes of heat or cold and because these medications are produced within living cell systems, no two batches are completely identical. Biologics used in IBD target areas of the immune system that are believed to cause inflammation. They are also used for a variety of other illnesses like cancer, arthritis, and psoriasis.

Biologics can be given as an injection into the stomach or thighs, or as an intravenous infusion into a vein.

Because these drugs are proteins, the body may reject them by producing antibodies, proteins that fight the biologic. It is important not to miss doses of the drug for this reason. If there is a longer time interval than planned between doses of the drug, the body can start rejecting it. If the body rejects it, allergic reactions such as skin rashes, shortness of breath, and chest pain can occur. In addition, the medication will lose its effectiveness for treating IBD. Physicians can check the blood levels of the drug itself and the antibodies, from time to time. This allows dosing to be tailored to the individual patient, especially if it appears that efficacy is wearing off and symptoms are appearing close to the injection/infusion.

There are currently four different classes of biologics available, anti-tumor necrosis factor (anti-TNFs), Vedolizumab (Entyvio), Ustekinumab (Stelara), and Risankizumab (Skyrizi). They target different areas of the immune cascade.

Biosimilars are biologic agents that are engineered to be highly similar to the original FDA approved biologic agent and are generally cheaper than the brand name. These biosimilars are as effective as the original agent and can be used interchangeably. We know this from many studies both in the United States and in Europe. There are currently biosimilars available for Remicade and Humira. Very often, the insurance company dictates which biologic can be prescribed for a patient based on what they have on their formulary (Table 5.1).

Table 5.1 Major characteristics of the currently available biologics

	Anti-TNF and biosimilars (Remicade, Humira, Cimzia, Inflectra)	Vedolizumab (Entyvio)	Ustekinumab (Stelara)	Risankizumab (Skyrizi)
Action	Blocks tumor necrosis factor (TNF)	Blocks integrins	Blocks interleukin 12 and 23	Blocks interleukin 23
Effects	More generalized effects	Selective to the gut	Acts on gut and skin	Acts on gut and skin
Used for	UC and CD. Rheumatoid arthritis, psoriasis, ankylosing spondylitis	UC and CD	UC and CD, psoriasis, and psoriatic arthritis	CD, psoriasis, and psoriatic arthritis
How it's given	*Remicade/Inflectra:* Intravenous infusions: Induction at 0,2,6 weeks, maintenance infusion every 8 weeks *Humira* (self-administered injection): Induction 0 week 160 mg, 2 weeks later 80 mg, then 40 mg every other week in prefilled syringe *Cimzia* (only for CD, self-administered injection): Induction: 400 mg injection on weeks 0, 2, 4, then Maintenance 400 mg injection every 4 weeks	Intravenous infusion: Induction at 0,2,6 weeks and then maintenance Intravenous infusion every 8 weeks	Induction with a single intravenous infusion Then maintenance with self-administered injections every 8 weeks	Induction with 3 intravenous infusions, 0,2,6 weeks, followed by self-administered injections every 2 months
Pre-infusion testing	Need to check hepatitis and TB blood tests before starting	Need to check hepatitis and TB blood tests before starting	Need to check hepatitis and TB blood tests before starting	Need to check hepatitis and TB blood tests before starting

Side Effects of Biologics

There are many potential side effects of biologics. Some of the well-known ones are listed below.

Allergic reactions: Shortness of breath, itching and skin rashes, joint pains, and chest pain.

Increased susceptibility to infections: Particularly upper respiratory tract infections but any infection can worsen with a biologic agent. It is best to hold the medication when there is active infection with fever, until it has resolved, after checking with your doctor. Patients are always checked for silent TB and hepatitis prior to initiation of biologics.

Worsening of other illnesses: Other illnesses can be worsened by some of these drugs including rheumatological, neurological, and cardiac conditions. Multiple sclerosis and congestive heart failure are contraindications to treatment with biologics. It is therefore important to ensure that your gastroenterologist is informed about all medical conditions that you may have.

Cancer risk: There is also concern of new lymphoma and reactivation of preexisting cancer in some patients. This appears to be mostly with anti-TNFs especially when used in combination with an immunomodulator. This is rare but should be discussed with your physician before starting a biologic.

It is important to let your physician know should you have any new symptoms or concerns after or before starting a biologic agent.

Duration of Treatment

Biologic agents are induction and maintenance drugs, and therefore must be initiated for long term in order to maintain efficacy and prevent allergic reactions and rejection of the medication. There are some patients who have been on these medications for many years and remained in remission. In specific instances, there may be an effort to stop the medications (de-escalation), but this must be weighed against the risk of developing antibodies and therefore, losing the medication for future use. Discontinuing a biologic should be undertaken with shared decision-making between the patient and the physician.

Steroids

Steroids are the oldest drugs available for use in IBD. They have a direct anti-inflammatory action and work fast. They are used to bring inflammation under control fast but should never be used as a long-term maintenance treatment, because of serious side effects. Long-term side effects are many and include bone loss and fractures, high blood sugar, cataracts, predisposition to infections, skin thinning, and weight gain.

They are used predominantly for UC, to bring a flare of colitis under control, but can also be used for CD. Steroids are administered orally for milder disease, and intravenously in the hospital for more severe disease. They should not be stopped abruptly, but rather tapered down, in order to prevent withdrawal symptoms.

Prednisone is an oral drug usually given at a dose of 40 mg or 60 mg orally for a period of time, usually a week, and then tapered down. The regimen used for tapering will depend on the severity of illness, and presence of other illnesses such as diabetes, as well as physician and patient preference.

Budesonide is a milder oral steroid that works "locally" in the intestines. It can be used to bring milder disease under control and has less side effects than prednisone. Budesonide is sold under the trade name of Entocort for treatment of ileitis. Budesonide that is coated for release in the colon alone, goes under the name of Uceris and can be used for the treatment of colitis.

Neither of these drugs should be used as long-term maintenance to prevent inflammation.

There are steroid enemas and foams that can be used for treatment of rectal or rectosigmoid inflammation as well. Hydrocortisone creams and suppositories can be used for the treatment of hemorrhoids.

Steroid creams may be used for the treatment of skin manifestations of IBD under the direction of a dermatologist. Steroid eyedrops may be used for treatment of inflammations of the eye under the direction of an ophthalmologist.

Immunomodulators

6-Mercaptopurine(6-MP)/Azathioprine (AZA)

These are older drugs, first used for the treatment of IBD in the early 1980s. They are oral medications that act on the immune system to modulate and reduce inflammation. They are also used for the treatment of certain types of leukemia, after kidney transplants to prevent rejection of the transplanted organ, and other autoimmune illnesses.

Azathioprine is the precursor of 6-MP. These drugs are administered orally, and the dose may be increased over a period of months to achieve remission. The mode of action is slow, and full effect can take anywhere from 4 months to a year.

These medications can cause a little nausea for the first few weeks and are therefore best taken at night. There can be potentially serious drug interactions with other medications, such as allopurinol, so it is important to inform your doctor about any other medications you may be taking.

They can have potentially serious but rare side effects, some of which are listed in Table 5.2.

Table 5.2 Side effects of 6-MP/AZA

Side effect	Symptom and tests to evaluate
Low hemoglobin (anemia)	Tiredness, shortness of breath (CBC)
Reduced white cell count	Fever, increased risk of infections (CBC)
Liver inflammation	Abdominal pain, jaundice (hepatic function panel)
Pancreas inflammation	Abdominal pain (amylase, lipase)
Allergic reaction	Hives, skin rashes, shortness of breath
Reduced platelets	Increased bleeding and bruising (CBC)
Hair loss	Hair loss (lab tests)

Monitoring: Blood levels of the enzyme that breaks the medication down are typically checked before starting 6-MP/AZA, and levels of other chemicals may be checked during the course of treatment in order to optimize the dose and prevent side effects. Your physician will order regular lab work such as CBC, hepatic function, and chemistries, to monitor for any evidence of inflammation in any of the other organs as listed above, because if the medication is reduced or stopped, the inflammation will often reverse. Any new or unusual symptoms such as abdominal pain, fatigue, nausea, or vomiting should be reported to your physician.

Methotrexate (MTx)

This is also an old drug, used more commonly to treat arthritis. It can be used to treat CD, but in ulcerative colitis, the evidence is lacking for effectiveness. It is more commonly used in combination with a biologic agent in order to increase the efficacy of the biologic and to prevent rejection of it. It can help to prevent allergic reactions to biologics.

MTx can be administered orally or by an injection, once per week. It has many potential side effects including liver and lung problems and can cause abnormalities in the fetus if a pregnant woman takes it. It is therefore absolutely contraindicated in pregnant women. It should be used with caution in any young woman who has the potential to become pregnant. If it is prescribed for a young woman, adequate birth control should be used.

Targeted Small Molecules

These are small molecules that are taken orally and target specific areas of the immune system. Although they are oral medications, that does not mean that they are mild or safer than biologics and immunomodulators. They can all cause problems with the heart, blood clotting, liver enzymes elevations, cholesterol elevations and infections, particularly shingles. Patients should have baseline blood tests drawn. If cholesterol is elevated, it should be treated. All patients should also be vaccinated with the shingles vaccine prior to beginning these medications. The currently available shingles vaccine is inactivated and safe to use even with immunomodulation. Close monitoring is required.

Tofacitinib (Xeljanz)

This is a pill (Janus Kinase inhibitor) that is used to treat UC patients who have failed other therapies. It is also used for the treatment of different types of arthritis and may be a good choice for patients who have both illnesses. It is administered orally at 10 mg twice a day and stopped after 2 months if it doesn't work. If it does work, the dose is reduced after 2 months to 5 mg twice daily for maintenance.

Potentially serious side effects include infections, heart disease, blood clots, increase in cholesterol, and perforation of the bowel. Cholesterol levels are checked prior to starting and followed after starting the medication and close clinical follow-up is required.

Upadacitinib (Rinvoq)

This is a Janus Kinase inhibitor administered as a once daily pill. It is indicated for the treatment of moderately to severely active ulcerative colitis in adults who have failed or had an inadequate response or intolerance to anti TNF agents. It is also indicated for arthritis, and severe eczema. The recommended induction dose for UC is 45 mg daily for 8 weeks, and maintenance is 15 mg daily. The medication is usually discontinued if it is ineffective after 8 weeks. Again, it can cause serious side effects including infections, heart disease, blood clots, increase in cholesterol. Lab testing will be checked on a regular basis and any new symptoms should be reported to your physician.

Ozanimod (Zeposia)

This is also an oral agent (S1P inhibitor) that targets the immune system and is approved for the treatment of ulcerative colitis as well as multiple sclerosis. It is contraindicated in patients who have had a heart attack, stroke, heart failure, or taking certain medications. It can also increase susceptibility to infections particularly shingles, so patients should be vaccinated against it. It may also cause elevation of liver enzymes, eye problems, neurological side effects, and respiratory side effects. Your physician will monitor you for all of these potential side effects and will discontinue the medication if they do occur. Lab work will also be closely monitored.

The medication is titrated and is in the form of a starter pack which makes titration easy to follow, over a 7-day period. It is then administered as a maintenance dose with a once daily pill.

Antibiotics

Antibiotics are sometimes used for the treatment of IBD. Ciprofloxacin and Flagyl have been used for many years, sometimes to treat infections, and sometimes because of their mild anti-inflammatory properties in CD. When there is very severe inflammation of the intestine or a collection of pus (abscess), antibiotics are prescribed orally or intravenously. Flagyl is used for the treatment of perianal fistulas and inflammation of a rectal pouch. It can be used at a low dose in the long term especially for perianal fistulas. Side effects of flagyl include a change in taste and neuropathies which can produce pins and needles in hands and feet. Side effects of Cipro include problems with joints. If any unusual symptoms occur, the physician should be informed, and the medication discontinued.

Sometimes patients with Crohn's disease and narrowing of the small intestine develop overgrowth of bad bacteria, called small intestinal bacterial overgrowth (SIBO). This can cause abdominal pain, flatulence, bloating, and a change in bowel habit. It is typically diagnosed with a breath test: a sugary drink is consumed and then you blow into a bag. Hydrogen and methane are measured. It can be treated with antibiotics which include Cipro and Flagyl, or rifaximin (Xifaxan). Unfortunately, SIBO tends to recur and may have to be treated multiple times.

Chapter 6
Complementary Therapies for IBD

There are numerous alternative options advertised and touted in social media and the internet for the treatment of, or as complementary to standard therapies. In standard medicine, medications must be proven effective, with minimal or statistically acceptable side effects, through randomized control trials (RCT) before they are approved by the FDA for general use by the public. In a RCT, the medication is compared to a placebo (a treatment that has no active properties such as a sugar pill) while the prescriber and patient are blinded to the drug. In this way, it is possible to determine if the medication in question really works. It does away with potential bias on the part of the patient or the prescribing physician. The problem with alternative therapies is that most of these treatments have not been subjected to, or have not been proven to be effective through rigorous randomized controlled trials. Similarly, dosing regimens and potential side effects are not well known either. They are not regulated by the FDA which adds to confusion for patients who rely on advertisers claims of efficacy.

Probiotics

These are live microorganisms that, when consumed (or sometimes when applied to the body), can supplement the microbiome and have health benefits. They are most commonly bacteria but can also be fungi. There are millions of microorganisms within the GI tract; some have significant health benefits and are important for the proper functioning of the body, while some can be harmful. This community of microorganisms that live in or on us is called the microbiome. The sum total of bacteria, fungi, and viruses in the gut is called the gut microbiome. The microbiome was first studied through the Human Microbiome Project supported by the National Institute of Health (NIH). Scientists are studying the association and links between the microbiome and many diseases and also looking into ways to treat diseases by

R. Rajapakse, *Crohn's Disease and Ulcerative Colitis*, https://doi.org/10.1007/978-3-031-45407-3_6

altering the microbiome, predominantly by ingestion of probiotics. It is believed that the microbiome functions almost like a separate organ, and the microorganisms have numerous beneficial as well as deleterious effects.

In the US, it is estimated that probiotics are the third most commonly used dietary supplement after vitamins and minerals.

How Do They Work?

There are several mechanisms postulated:

- Increased numbers of good bacteria will keep down the numbers of harmful bacteria
- They help with digestion by producing enzymes
- They produce substances that are beneficial to the body
- They enhance the immune system of the gut thus enabling it to respond better to noxious stimuli

The most common bacteria in probiotics are lactobacillus and bifidobacterium, while the most common yeast is Saccharomyces boulardii. Many probiotic preparations are sold as nutritional supplements and are therefore not regulated by the US Food and Drug Administration (FDA).

A great deal of research has been done on the use of probiotics for various conditions with mixed results. The current thinking is that adding a probiotic to standard therapy in UC can be helpful. This is especially so in pouchitis (inflammation of the ileal pouch created after a colectomy). In CD, the benefit is more questionable.

Side Effects: Probiotics are generally safe. They may sometimes cause gas and bloating.

Prebiotics

Prebiotics are plant fibers that are not digested and absorbed, remain in the gut, and help bacteria grow: they are nutrition for the good bacteria, so to speak.

They have other potential beneficial effects:

- Improve calcium absorption and therefore bone health
- Decrease spikes in blood sugar
- Ferment and breakdown food faster, promoting elimination and reducing constipation
- Keep gut cells healthy

The best way to get prebiotics is from whole foods, and there are many foods, such as fruits, vegetables, and whole grains, that qualify in this category. Good sources of prebiotics include chicory root, dandelion greens, apples, garlic, onions, bananas, and whole oats. Sometimes prebiotics are added to foods like breakfast cereals. When you see substances like galacto-oligosaccharides, fructo-oligosaccharides, chicory fiber, and inulin on labels, these are prebiotics.

However, too many prebiotics can cause gas and bloating. They should be avoided or used only in small quantities in patients with small intestinal bacterial overgrowth (SIBO) because they can worsen the condition and symptoms of gas and bloating.

Cannabinoids (Marijuana)

Marijuana has become very popular for managing a wide range of illnesses. Cannabinoid receptors are found both in the nervous system and in the gut, CB1 and CB2. Activation of gut receptors can help to modulate pain and function of the GI tract.

The two active substances in marijuana are tetrahydrocannabinol (THC) and cannabidiol (CBD). THC is responsible for the neurological and mood enhancing effects while both THC and CBD can help to reduce pain in the gut.

Although researchers are studying the effects of both compounds on IBD, there is no evidence yet that they reduce inflammation and therefore help to treat IBD. They can, however, help some patients with symptom management.

The number one reason that IBD patients use cannabis is to control abdominal pain. Unfortunately, regular cannabis use can mask inflammation, because symptoms may improve or be less troublesome, without a decrease in inflammation. Sometimes cannabinoids can cause abdominal pain and nausea, confusing the situation further.

Caution should be exercised with excessive use. Chronic and excessive use of cannabis can lead to decreased mental sharpness, nausea, vomiting, cyclic vomiting, and possibly decreased fertility. There is in fact some evidence that CD patients who used a lot of cannabis, for greater than 6 months, had a higher chance of requiring surgery.

Curcumin (Turmeric)

Curcumin is derived from the root of the curcumin plant which is from the same family as ginger. It is a bright yellow root. It is popular in Asia where it is used as a spice in food and in a variety of herbal remedies. In animal studies, curcumin appears to have a beneficial effect on intestinal inflammation, but only when used in its purest form. It can be considered as a complement to currently available standard therapies but there is insufficient data in the medical literature to recommend routine use.

Omega 3 Fatty Acids

Omega 3 fatty acids are polyunsaturated fats that have an important function in the body. The human body cannot produce the amount of Omega 3s that are needed for proper functioning; therefore, they are an essential nutrient. They are also important for maintaining a healthy colon and are usually derived from transformation of fat in foods by bacteria in the gut. The best food sources of omega-3 fatty acids include certain types of fish, ground flaxseed, walnuts, and edamame beans. Fish is overall the best source of Omega 3s, and out of most fish, salmon and mackerel seem to have the highest concentration. Omega 3 supplements provide the same fatty acids in pill form at high concentrations.

Experimental studies have not shown a benefit in CD. The results in UC are mixed with some studies showing a benefit with large doses and others showing no benefit compared to placebo.

Omega 3 supplements are generally safe, but can interfere with some prescription medications, and increase your risk of bleeding. They can also have unpleasant side effects such as causing a fishy breath odor when taken in high concentrations. Always check with your physician before starting any over-the-counter supplement.

Exercise

Exercise is good for overall health, particularly of the heart and lungs but it also has mood elevating effects. Exercise is well known to decrease mortality in the general population, likely through a reduction in heart disease and cancer. In IBD, exercise has been linked to an improved quality of life, improved bone health, and less flares in both UC and CD. Potential reasons for the benefit include release of substances during exercise that may reduce inflammation, improve immune function, and repair cells.

There are no guidelines for exercise in patients with IBD. However, to promote and maintain health, joint guidelines from the American Heart Association and the American Academy of sports medicine recommend either:

1. Moderate intensity aerobic exercise (you can talk but not sing during exercise) for a minimum of 30 min 5 days per week or
2. Vigorous intensity physical activity (you can't say more than a few words without pausing for breath) for 20 min, 3 days per week for people between the ages of 18 and 65 years of age

In conclusion, use of complementary therapies is very common in IBD. Most of these therapies do not have strong evidence to indicate that they really work, particularly not on their own. However, many of these modalities are generally safe and may produce some improvement in symptoms when used in combination with standard treatments. Always check with your physician prior to using complementary therapies in IBD.

Chapter 7
Nutrition in IBD

Many patients with IBD are confused about what to eat and whether something they are eating caused or is contributing to their illness. There has been a lot of research into this area including the use of very defined diets, but no specific diet has been shown to prevent or treat IBD. However, some dietary modifications can be helpful in reducing symptoms. It is useful to keep a diary, with a record of dates, foods consumed, and symptoms for a period of time. That way dietary triggers and patterns can be identified, and those foods avoided, because one's memory can be fickle. It is important not to restrict foods randomly unless they cause symptoms, because it is important to ensure a balanced diet.

IBD can lead to malnutrition, more so in CD than in UC. Malnutrition is more common in CD than in UC because nutrient absorption occurs in the small intestine. If there is inflammation in the small intestine, it can lead to decreased absorption of nutrients. This is especially important in children because it can cause inadequate growth and short stature. Increased losses of fluids and electrolytes from the intestines can occur with diarrhea and should be supplemented with drinks containing electrolytes such as Gatorade, Pedialyte, and Powerade. Deficiencies of vitamins and minerals can occur as outlined in other parts of this book.

Active inflammation anywhere in the body can lead to pain, loss of appetite, and weight loss.

General Dietary Guidelines

According to the CDC guidelines for the general public, it is important to eat foods that promote health and manage weight. This means having a wide variety of different foods and colors which automatically then boosts nutrition. The dietary guidelines for Americans 2020 to 2025 from the CDC emphasize fruits, vegetables, whole grains, fat-free or low-fat milk, a variety of protein foods such as sea foods, lean

R. Rajapakse, *Crohn's Disease and Ulcerative Colitis*, https://doi.org/10.1007/978-3-031-45407-3_7

meats, poultry, eggs, legumes, nuts, and seeds. It also emphasizes a diet low in added sugars, sodium, saturated fats, trans fats, and cholesterol and must stay within the daily caloric needs depending on age, sex, and activity level.

The average woman requires about 2000 calories per day, and the average man requires about 2500 calories per day. This varies depending on age and level of activity. The dietary guidelines for Americans (Department of human and health services) recommend that an adult's total daily calories come from 45 to 65% carbohydrates, 10 to 30% protein, and 20 to 35% fat. The best carbohydrates are complex carbohydrates (such as whole grains). Refined carbohydrates such as white flour and sugar are best avoided as they cause rapid fluctuations in blood glucose and predispose to obesity. When considering proteins, it is important to consider the source of protein. Lean meat such as chicken breast, and fish are preferable to red meat. Plant proteins can also provide essential amino acids. In terms of fat consumption, it is best to consume polyunsaturated, monounsaturated, and omega-3 fatty acids and avoid saturated and trans fats.

These guidelines must be modified for IBD patients again depending on age, gender, and activity level as well as disease process and presence or absence of complications. For example, a patient with Crohn's disease and a chronic narrowing of the intestinal tract would need to limit fiber in the diet in order to prevent intestinal obstruction.

In assessing weight, the best measure, though not perfect, is the body mass index (BMI). This calculation can be obtained via a BMI calculator online, by entering your weight, height, and sex.

- *BMI < 18.5*: underweight
- *BMI 18.5–24.9*: healthy weight
- *BMI 25.0–29.9*, overweight
- *BMI > 30.0* obese

The BMI should only be used as an indicator and is not diagnostic of body fatness or the health of any individual person, particularly in patients with IBD.

Potential Nutritional Deficiencies

Vitamin B12

This vitamin is absorbed in the terminal ileum (the last part of the small intestine). Therefore, if there is inflammation in the terminal ileum or removal of this area surgically, B12 deficiency can result. B12 deficiency usually begins without any symptoms and may only be picked up on routine blood tests. However, it can produce anemia which in turn can cause tiredness, lack of vitality, and shortness of breath and/or chest pain on exertion. Neurological symptoms such as pins and needles in the hands or feet or problems with balance can occur with more advanced deficiency. Treatment has to be with injections of B12 or preparations that dissolve under the tongue because regular oral vitamin supplements will not be absorbed. Vitamin B12 is only found in animal-based products. Therefore, vegans, especially those with CD, are more prone to vitamin B12 deficiency and should pay particular attention to consuming fortified foods or a separate vitamin pill.

Good sources of vitamin B12 include the following:

- Eggs
- Beef, liver, chicken
- Fortified breakfast cereals
- Milk, cheese, yoghurt
- Fish, shellfish (e.g., tuna, salmon, sole, trout, shrimps, clams)
- Yeast, yeast spreads, and fortified foods

Folate

Deficiency of this vitamin can occur with the use of certain medications such as sulfasalazine or methotrexate. Therefore, any patient receiving these medications should also receive folate supplementation at 1 mg per day. Folate deficiency can cause anemia in adults, and neurological problems in the fetus, if a woman is pregnant. That is why all prenatal vitamins contain folate. Folate is found in a wide variety of foods. The US Food and Drug administration (FDA) requires the addition of folate to many commonly consumed foods.

Good sources of folate include the following:

- Green leafy vegetables like spinach, lettuce, brussels sprouts, and broccoli
- Beans and lentils
- Whole grains (brown rice, buckwheat, bulghur)
- Seafood
- Eggs

Interestingly some patients who have small intestinal bacterial overgrowth (SIBO) have elevated levels of blood folate due to production of folate by bacteria. This can act as a clue to the diagnosis.

Vitamins A, D, E, K

These vitamins are absorbed in the small intestine bound to fats and are considered "fat soluble" vitamins. Therefore, if there is extensive small intestinal inflammation or surgical resection in CD, these vitamins may become deficient. Deficiency can lead to bone loss, skin problems, eye problems, bleeding problems, and problems with the nervous system. Patients with extensive surgery or inflammation of the small intestines should take vitamin supplements.

Good sources of vitamin D

- Milk and dairy products
- Oily fish
- Sunlight

Good sources of vitamin A
Vegetables with carotene like carrots, sweet potatoes, squash (orange vegetables)

- Cantaloupes
- Apricots
- Leafy vegetables like kale, spinach, and collard greens

Good sources of vitamin E

- Leafy greens like spinach, swiss chard, and kale.
- Bell peppers
- Asparagus

Good sources of vitamin K

- Leafy green vegetables like kale, spinach, collard greens
- Brussels sprouts
- Broccoli
- Asparagus

Magnesium

Chronic diarrhea or fluid losses through a fistula can result in magnesium deficiency. Magnesium is important for regulating muscle and nerve function, ensuring stable blood sugar levels and for the production of protein, bone, and DNA. Magnesium deficiency may initially be asymptomatic, but can produce many symptoms including loss of appetite, nausea, fatigue, muscle weakness, and heart arrhythmias. If there is a deficiency, foods high in magnesium should be consumed, and oral magnesium supplements should be taken.

Good sources of magnesium include the following:

- Pumpkin seeds and chia seeds
- Nuts like almonds, cashews, peanuts
- Spinach
- Bananas

Zinc

Zinc is an essential mineral and is very important for cell metabolism. It also enhances immune function, wound healing, and DNA synthesis. It is involved in the sense of taste. Extensive surgery or inflammation in CD can result in decreased absorption or loss of zinc. The effect of zinc deficiency varies. In infants and children, diarrhea is a common sign and it can also lead to impaired growth and loss of appetite. Zinc deficiency in older adults can cause impaired wound healing and changes in cognitive and psychological function. Skin rashes and altered taste sensation may occur as well. Oral supplements are available.

Good sources of zinc include the following:

- Meats
- Fish
- Legumes like beans and lentils
- Seeds like pumpkin and sesame seeds

Calcium

Calcium is required to maintain strong bones. It is the most abundant mineral in the body because it is contained in bones. It is what gives bones and teeth their structure and hardness. Calcium is also required for muscles and nerve function, blood vessels, and hormones. Calcium deficiency can occur for a variety of reasons.

Decreased intake: Dairy intolerance (lactose intolerance) can lead to avoidance of dairy products which are high in calcium.

Decreased absorption of calcium: Inflammation of the small intestine or resection of parts of it in CD, can result in reduced absorption of calcium.

Decreased vitamin D: Vitamin D is important for the absorption of calcium and therefore deficiency of vitamin D either due to lack of sun or insufficient dietary intake can result in calcium deficiency.

Kidney disease: Diseased kidneys cause increased loss of calcium in the urine causing deficiency.

Certain medications such as steroids can result in calcium deficiency. Calcium deficiency can lead to osteoporosis and an increased risk of fractures. Although in the general population, this is more common in women particularly postmenopausal women, in the IBD population it can affect men as well.

Supplementation with oral calcium or vitamin D may be required. Some calcium supplements can cause gas and bloating, especially those containing carbonate (calcium carbonate). Trial and error is useful in finding a preparation that is tolerated.

Good dietary sources of calcium include the following:

- Dairy products like milk, yoghurt, and cheese.
- Sardines and canned salmon.

- Legumes like beans and lentils.
- Leafy greens like kale and spinach.

Potassium

Potassium is an essential nutrient; it is present in all body tissues and cells and is vital in maintaining optimal cellular and tissue conditions. Potassium and sodium are closely linked. Chronic diarrhea and vomiting can cause a lack of potassium due to increased loss either in the stool or in the vomit. When potassium deficiency is mild, it may only cause fatigue, muscle weakness, and constipation, but when it is more severe, it can cause heart arrhythmia, muscle weakness, and problems with breathing. Severe potassium deficiency can be life threatening. Potassium levels are checked on routine blood panels. It can be supplemented with diet and oral tablets.

Good sources of potassium include the following:

- Bananas
- Dried fruits like raisins and apricots
- Potatoes with skin
- Acorn squash
- Lentils
- Avocado
- Milk, chicken, fish

Iron

Iron is used to make hemoglobin, which is the protein that carries oxygen, found in red blood cells. Iron is also required to make hormones. The amount of iron required depends on age, gender, and diet. Causes of iron deficiency include the following:

- Iron loss due to bleeding, especially in active UC. This is compounded in women with heavy menses.
- Decreased small intestinal absorption in CD with small intestinal inflammation or after surgical resection of small intestine.
- Decreased iron intake due to pain or illness.

Iron deficiency causes anemia, which can result in weakness, shortness of breath, and low energy. Supplementation with diet, oral tablets, and intravenous infusions are all available. Iron supplements are available as ferrous sulfate, ferrous gluconate, ferric citrate, and ferric sulfate. The supplements have to be kept out of reach of children as they are a cause of fatal poisoning in children due to accidental overdose. Iron supplements can cause GI side effects, so it is recommended that you try a small amount of preparation and switch to a different one if it causes a problem. If a patient cannot tolerate oral iron or there is significant difficulty with absorption, or if the anemia is severe, iron can also be given intravenously. Intravenous iron infusions will replace iron much faster than oral iron. This is done in a doctor's office or clinic through an intravenous infusion and can take several hours. It may need to be repeated several times until adequate blood iron levels are all obtained. Side effects of intravenous iron are minimal but can include allergic type reactions. This is why the patient is monitored during the iron infusion. Iron levels start to normalize about 1–4 weeks after infusion.

Good dietary sources of iron include the following:

- Beef or chicken liver
- Shellfish like oysters, mussels
- Beef
- Chicken
- Fish like haddock and tuna
- Fortified foods
- White beans, lentils, spinach, nuts, raisins, peas

Diet may have to be changed depending on whether there is a flare or not and whether there are complications such as intestinal narrowing or fistulae. It is important to discuss nutrition and diet with your doctor. The above recommendations should only be used as a general guide.

Nutritional Side Effects of Medications

Sulfasalazine: Folate deficiency (supplement)
   Methotrexate: Folate deficiency(supplement)
   Steroids: Calcium deficiency(supplement)

Crohn's Flare, General Recommendations

Always discuss the best dietary measures with your physician. In general, when Crohn's is flaring, it is best to have a low fiber diet (see Appendix). This is especially important if there is narrowing of the intestine and there are symptoms suggestive of obstruction or impending obstruction such as abdominal distension, nausea, vomiting, failure to pass gas or stool and abdominal pain. If symptoms are severe, it is important to seek medical attention right away. If less severe and partial blockage is suspected, a clear liquid diet is indicated. A clear liquid diet consists of liquids you can see through such as plain Jell-o, water, broth, tea/coffee without milk, and clear drinks. If diarrhea is a predominant symptom, it is important to keep up hydration with electrolytes: Gatorade, Pedialyte, and vitamin water are good options.

Even without a history of dairy intolerance, following a low dairy diet may be helpful during a flare because when the lining of the intestine is inflamed, the ability to digest milk products becomes reduced. When it is not digested, milk is fermented by bacteria in the gut causing gas, bloating, and diarrhea, thus exacerbating Crohn's symptoms.

Smaller, more frequent meals are preferable to less frequent large meals.

Nutrient dense foods should be chosen. Processed foods should be avoided. Limit the intake of saturated and trans fats, cholesterol, added sugar, salt, and alcohol.

If an adequate food intake is not possible, consider taking a nutritional supplement such as ensure or boost.

UC Flare, General Recommendations

Although a low fiber diet is not medically necessary, it may help to relieve abdominal discomfort, gas, and bloating. Frequent small meals are recommended with nutrient dense foods. Avoid substances that can increase stool frequency such as caffeinated drinks (coffee/tea/soda/chocolate), fruit juices, and sugar free substances (aspartame, sucralose, maltitol, and sorbitol). Drink plenty of fluids and supplement with electrolyte drinks such as Gatorade/ Pedialyte and vitamin water. Consider a nutritional supplement if dietary intake is poor.

Once the flare is improving and symptoms are improving, regular foods can be re-introduced.

Chapter 8
Surgical Options for Crohn's and Colitis

Surgery plays different roles in UC and CD. Since UC affects only the colon, removal of the colon, a colectomy, is potentially a cure. On the other hand, since CD can affect the entire GI tract, removal of portions of inflamed gut does not cure Crohn's because it can recur in other parts of the remaining intestine.

Surgery should not be viewed as a last resort, and ideally consultation with a surgeon should be made before there is an urgent need for it. A surgical option should be used before there are long lasting and debilitating complications of the disease. Therefore, timing of surgery is important and should be determined through a multidisciplinary approach involving the gastroenterologist, the surgeon, other involved physicians and, of course, the patient. It is best to try and avoid an emergency surgery if at all possible.

Surgery in UC

The first line of treatment for UC is medications as outlined in Chap. 5. The choice of medication will depend on the extent and severity of inflammation, insurance issues, other medical conditions, and patient preference.

Indications for surgery in UC

- Failure of medical treatment with ongoing chronic symptoms.
- Side effects to available medications.
- Precancerous lesions (called dysplasia) in the colon or a diagnosis of colon cancer.
- Severe uncontrolled rectal bleeding.
- Colonic perforation (hole in the wall of the colon).
- Severe enlargement of the colon (toxic megacolon).

© The Author(s), under exclusive license to Springer Nature
Switzerland AG 2023
R. Rajapakse, *Crohn's Disease and Ulcerative Colitis*,
https://doi.org/10.1007/978-3-031-45407-3_8

Surgical Options in UC

1. Removal of the entire colon and rectum with an ileostomy (see Fig. 8.1).

   In this type of surgery, the entire colon and rectum are removed. This surgery can be performed laparoscopically or robotically, instead of open. The anus is closed, and the small intestine is brought out onto the skin, usually on the right side of the abdomen, in the form of a stoma, called an ileostomy. A bag is attached to the stoma, which collects stool. This bag has to be emptied whenever it fills, about 3–4 times per day depending on diet. This surgery is potentially curative because there is no colon left.

   Problems:

   (a) The stoma can become irritated or can twist. If twisting occurs, it may have to be revised
   (b) Patient may have difficulty adapting to life with a bag
   (c) Sometimes the diagnosis of colitis is unclear or has to be revised in which case inflammation can occur in the small intestine

2. Removal of the entire colon and rectum and creation of a "fake rectum": J Pouch (Ileal Pouch Anal Anastomosis, IPAA)

   In this surgery, the colon and rectum are removed, and a pouch is created in the rectum using small bowel (Fig. 8.2).

   The surgery may be done in up to 3 stages depending on many factors related to the disease, the patient and the surgeon, but is usually performed in two.

   In a one-stage procedure, the colon and rectum are removed, and the ileum is made into a J-shaped pouch and connected to the anal canal. This is not done

Fig. 8.1 Ileostomy after total colectomy

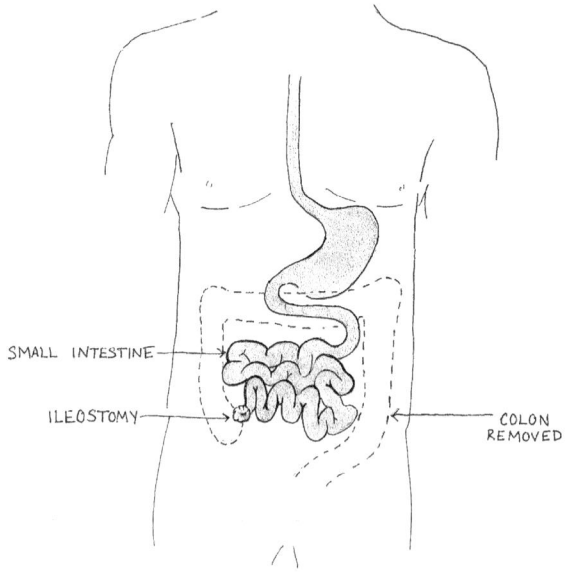

SMALL INTESTINE

ILEOSTOMY

COLON REMOVED

Fig. 8.2 Ileal pouch anal anastomosis (IPAA) ("J" pouch)

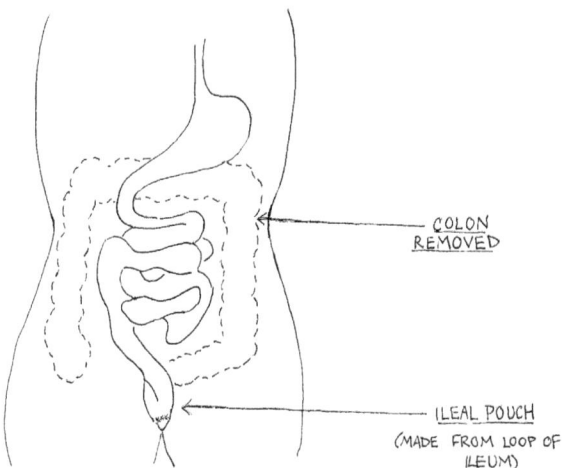

COLON REMOVED

ILEAL POUCH
(MADE FROM LOOP OF ILEUM)

often due to the risk of leakage from the anastomosis (the joined part) and infection.

In a two-stage procedure, the colon and rectum are removed, the ileum is made into a J-shaped pouch and connected to the anal canal, but a temporary ileostomy is created to allow the pouch to heal. A loop of small intestine is pulled through a small opening in the abdomen call a loop ileostomy, to allow waste to exit. A second surgery is required 8–12 weeks (about 3 months) later, once the pouch has healed, to reverse the temporary ileostomy, and allows waste products to pass through the IPAA and anus.

In a three-stage procedure, the first surgery removes the colon and creates the ileostomy: in the second surgery, the rectum is removed, and the ileum is formed into a pouch, and in the third surgery, the ileostomy is reversed, and the small intestine is reattached to the pouch. This is only recommended for patients who are in poor physical health, on high doses of steroids which increases risk, or if they needed emergency surgery for bleeding or a toxic colon.

The technical success rate for the pouch procedure is around 95% but complications can arise in about 15%. When it is successful, there is no longer urgency or bleeding.

Problems with the pouch:

(a) There are typically about 6 bowel movements/day although initially it can be as high as 12.
(b) Occasionally, the pouch may become inflamed, called pouchitis. This can be treated with medications.
(c) Pouch fistulas may require additional treatment.
(d) Pouch failure may require another surgery to recreate the pouch or to remove it and create a permanent ileostomy.
(e) Some male patients may develop sexual dysfunction due to nerve damage.
(f) Some female patients may develop infertility (approximately 25%).

3. Removal of most of the colon and joining (anastomosing) the ileum to the rectum (subtotal colectomy and ileorectal anastomosis). This may be performed
   under specific circumstances. It is not ideal because anorectal tissue is left behind
   and can still become inflamed causing bloody diarrhea and urgency. This area is
   also at risk for colon cancer and will need regular surveillance. The advantage is
   not requiring more extensive surgery to create an IPAA.

Surgical Options in CD

The first line of therapy for Crohn's disease is medication. Although Crohn's disease management has advanced with the introduction of biologic therapy and targeted small molecules, about half of patients with Crohn's disease still require
surgery within the first decade of diagnosis.

However, as mentioned previously, it is important to determine the optimal timing of surgery, especially in patients who have chronic strictures and narrowing,
inflamed masses or pus pockets called abscesses. Sometimes, early intervention
with surgery and then initiation of the appropriate therapy after surgery can result in
a better outcome than delaying surgery until there is malnutrition and extensive
chronic inflammation.

Indications for Surgery in CD

- Failure of medical treatment with worsening disease and inflammation
- Side effects to medication
- Complications

Complications Requiring Surgery in CD

1. **Stricture:** Obstruction of the intestine due to continued inflammation and scar
   tissue. Significant obstruction will cause abdominal pain, swelling, nausea, and
   vomiting, which may not respond to medical treatment. In this situation, the narrowed segment can be removed and the healthy tissue sewn back together. In
   many instances, this can be performed with a minimally invasive approach.
   Sometimes, instead of cutting out the affected part, the narrowed area can be
   opened up with a balloon or by means of diagonal suturing during surgery, called
   strictureplasty. Advanced endoscopist may be able to use a knife during an endoscopic procedure to open a narrowing as well, thus avoiding surgery.
2. **Abscesses:** Pus pockets, called abscesses, can occur within the abdomen or in
   the skin. They are a result of persistent inflammation spreading through the wall
   of the intestine, causing microscopic tears in the lining with leakage of gut contents and bacterial infection. If left untreated, this condition can become life
   threatening. Small abscesses may respond to antibiotic treatment alone, but

larger abscesses will require drainage. Drainage can be done by a radiologist using CT to guide the insertion of a needle, or by a surgeon.

3. **Fistulae.** When there is an abnormal connection between a loop of intestine and another loop of intestine or another organ, a fistula is said to have formed. Although these may sometimes close with medications (especially biologics), surgery is often required. This is especially so when the fistula is between the intestine and the vagina or bladder because it can cause recurrent infections of the urinary tract.

4. **Bleeding.** Major bleeding can occur if the inflammation and ulceration in the intestine spread through the intestinal wall into a blood vessel. This is rare when it occurs in CD. When this occurs, surgery is required to stop the bleeding.

5. **Dysplasia or cancer.** Patients with Crohn's of the small intestine are at risk for cancer and lymphoma of the small intestine. Crohn's of the colon can predispose to colon cancer. The risk depends on the extent and duration of inflammation. If there is cancer or early cancer (dysplasia), surgery is indicated to remove the affected part of the intestine.

6. **Perforation:** Spontaneous hole in the intestine. This is an emergency and requires surgery to fix.

The most important thing to remember with surgery for Crohn's disease is that surgery is not curative of Crohn's. Once the surgery has been completed, it is important to restart medication in order to prevent inflammation from recurring. The timing of medication in relation to surgery depends on the severity of inflammation, the presence or absence of complications, patient preference, and physician comfort. Sometimes it is preferable to start a biologic agent soon after the surgery. Another option is to perform periodic disease assessment with CT scans, MRIs, and colonoscopies, and to restart therapy as soon as there is any evidence of inflammation seen.

Postoperative Recurrence of Crohn's Disease

Because Crohn's disease recurs after surgery it is very important to monitor both clinically and with objective assessments. Clinical recurrence rate has been reported from 36 to 86% at 10 years, and endoscopic recurrence rates even higher and up to 70% within the first 6 months.

Several risk factors have been identified that make individuals at high or low risk after resection in Crohn's disease. These can be divided into patient-related, disease-related, and surgery-related risk factors:

The main patient-related risk factor is smoking. Studies have repeatedly identified the fact that smoking increases the risk of recurrence of Crohn's disease after surgery.

In terms of the disease itself, duration of Crohn's prior to the first surgery, history of previous surgery, extent of involvement, and presence of complications such as fistulas and narrowing all increase the risk of recurrence. Shorter duration of Crohn's prior to requiring the first surgery seems to increase the recurrence risk.

Surgery related-risk factors include the length of resection and the type of anastomosis, but these studies have not been consistent.

In high-risk patients, early intervention with medications is recommended in order to prevent more surgery.

Patients with Crohn's disease at lower risk for recurrence after surgery would be nonsmokers, no prior surgery, short strictures, and a long duration of illness prior to the first surgery. Even in the low-risk patient, it is recommended that they be monitored endoscopically every 6–12 months with colonoscopy, in order to determine when to begin and when to advance treatment. Stool studies for calprotectin can be followed together with the endoscopic findings.

In terms of medical treatment to prevent postoperative recurrence, only the anti-TNFs, 6 MP, and azathioprine have sufficient medical data to support routine use. The newer biologic agents do not have sufficient data as yet to recommend routine use for prevention of post-operative recurrence, but findings from sporadic data appear to be positive.

Chapter 9
Living with IBD

Like most other chronic illnesses, there is no cure for IBD as yet. Medications can be used to control inflammation and therefore symptoms, and reduce the risk of complications, but there is no medication that will cure it. Surgery may be required under certain circumstances and can be curative for UC but not for CD, as outlined elsewhere.

When the inflammation is under control, most patients can lead a full and normal life, forgetting sometimes about their disease. Some patients can have symptom free periods for many months or even years, off medication. However, in most instances, without medication, the inflammation eventually comes back. Sometimes within months, and sometimes within years.

It is very important to establish a good relationship with a physician who is familiar with IBD. Taking medications as prescribed is important, as is honesty and truthfulness with your doctor. An honest relationship is important in order to get the best possible care and outcome. If the symptoms themselves, or anxiety regarding symptoms, are affecting the patient's quality of life, it is important to convey this to the doctor.

It may seem unnecessary to take medication when there are no symptoms, but it is important to remember that taking maintenance medication as prescribed is important to prevent flares. (Similar to taking diabetic medication even when the blood sugar is low, or blood pressure medications even when blood pressure is controlled). It is because of the medication that the inflammation is controlled and therefore continuing the medication is vitally important.

When symptoms permit, it is important to continue daily life as normally as possible, including hobbies and exercise. Exercise is very important not only for general physical health but also for relaxation and mental well-being, as outlined elsewhere.

Sometimes Over the Counter (OTC) medications can help with symptom control (Table 9.1). You should always check with your physician before taking any OTC medications.

R. Rajapakse, *Crohn's Disease and Ulcerative Colitis*, https://doi.org/10.1007/978-3-031-45407-3_9

Table 9.1 Common GI symptoms and OTC meds that can help

Symptom	Medication
Gas and bloating	Simethicone (gas X), beano
Heartburn	Pepcid, Prilosec, Nexium, Mylanta, Maalox, TUMS
Constipation	MiraLAX, senna, Dulcolax, milk of magnesium, Colace
Hemorrhoids	Preparation H suppositories and ointment
Diarrhea	Imodium, peppermint supplement (IBgard)
Upper abdominal pain	Pepcid, Prilosec, Mylanta, Maalox
Lower abdominal cramps	Pepto-Bismol

Lifestyle Measures for Common GI Complaints

Heartburn

Heartburn is caused by gastroesophageal reflux: acid moving up from the stomach into the esophagus. The stomach is resistant to acid, but the esophagus is not. So, when acid refluxes into the esophagus, it causes a burning sensation, called heartburn. There are several foods that can trigger heartburn and should be avoided to prevent symptoms.

1. Caffeinated beverages like coffee, tea, soda, chocolate. Caffeine relaxes the lower esophagus and opens it up to allow acid to move up into esophagus.
2. Citrus fruits and juices: Orange, lemon, lime, grapefruit all have high acid and can worsen symptoms.
3. Tomatoes can affect the lower esophageal sphincter.
4. Fizzy drinks: These cause distension of the stomach and burping which allows movement of acid into the esophagus.
5. Fatty foods, alcohol, and smoking (nicotine): Also relax the lower esophageal sphincter and allow passage of acid up into the esophagus.

It is important that the last meal should be 4 h or more before lying down to allow enough time for the stomach to empty out. Lying down with a full stomach will allow food and acid to regurgitate up the esophagus, due to gravity. Sometimes a wedge under the mattress or wooden blocks under the head of the bed can be used to elevate the head of the bed, especially if there is a history of nighttime reflux.

If there is chronic heartburn, or any other symptoms associated with it, such as difficulty swallowing, painful swallowing, nausea, vomiting, or vomiting of blood, it is important to inform your physician who may prescribe a acid blocking medication. They may also recommend an upper endoscopy to rule out inflammation, precancerous changes (Barrett's esophagus) or Crohn's of the stomach which may affect the choice of treatment.

Gas/Bloating/Excessive Flatus

Excessive gas can occur due to ingested gas or due to fermentation of foods.

In order to decrease air swallowing, avoid chewing gum and sucking candy. Eat slowly and mindfully, chew food well, and avoid talking while eating. Avoid carbonated (fizzy) drinks. Avoid drinking through a straw as this allows sucking in excessive air as well.

It is important to know if you are lactose intolerant. Many patients who have gas and bloating, particularly with IBD, also have lactose intolerance. Undigested lactose in the intestine is fermented by bacteria to produce gas and diarrhea. Adherence to a lactose free diet or supplementing with lactaid pills (the missing enzyme) can help.

There are other foods that can increase gas production in the gut. Some food products are more prone to cause gas than others, and it is important to be able to identify them.

High Gas Foods
- Milk and milk products such as cheese, ice cream, and yoghurt (in lactose intolerant individuals).
- Onions.
- Beans (black beans, pinto beans, garbanzo, lentils, etc.).
- Cruciferous vegetables: Broccoli, cauliflower, brussels sprouts, cabbage.
- Sugar substitute alcohols like sorbitol.
- Prunes and prune juice.
- High carbohydrate foods like bagels and bread.

If gas and bloating persist in spite of careful dietary manipulation, it is important to inform your physician. Small intestinal bacterial overgrowth can cause similar symptoms especially in association with Crohn's narrowing and distention of the small intestine.

Lactose Intolerance

Lactose is a sugar found in dairy products derived from milk, such as milk itself, cheese, cream, yoghurt, ice cream, and butter. It is also found in many prepared and processed foods. Lactose intolerant people lack an enzyme, lactase, produced by the small intestine, that is used to digest lactose. Undigested lactose is fermented by bacteria in the gut producing abdominal discomfort, gas, bloating, and diarrhea. Lactose intolerance is not the same thing as having a food allergy to milk. In a food allergy, the person is allergic to certain constituents of milk. Lactose intolerance is a very common condition throughout the world. It is most common in Asian Americans, African Americans, Mexicans, and native Americans. It also tends to run in families. There are grades of lactose intolerance so that some people have severe intolerance, and others only have mild intolerance. Also, different dairy products have variable amounts of lactose. For example, Ice cream has large amount of lactose, while some hard cheeses and yoghurt have less. Therefore, not all dairy products will cause a problem in every lactose intolerant person. It is very important to read food labels. Lactose is often added to prepared foods such as bread, cereal, cake and cookie mixes, desserts, coffee creamer, and lunch meats. It is also added to many sauces, particularly pasta sauces. It is important to inform servers regarding lactose intolerance at restaurants because milk and milk products are used for thickening and flavoring of many different foods, particularly in Italian and French cuisine.

Symptoms of lactose intolerance vary from person to person but include gas, diarrhea, bloating, abdominal pain, and nausea. It is easy to see how some of the symptoms are very similar to the symptoms of Crohn's itself.

Lactose intolerance is often diagnosed by the patients themselves because they note abdominal discomfort and other symptoms whenever they consume dairy products. However, many lactose intolerant people don't know that they are, because they can consume some milk products without a problem. Reactions can also be delayed. Lactose intolerance can be definitively diagnosed through a lactose breath test. In this test, the patient is given a glass of milk to drink and then blows into a bag. The amount of hydrogen that comes out with the breath is measured. If it is really high, it implies that there is lactose intolerance.

Treatment for lactose intolerance includes avoidance of dairy products or the use of lactaid pills whenever dairy is consumed. Lactaid pills are available over the counter and contain the missing enzyme necessary to digest dairy. If dairy is being avoided due to lactose intolerance, it is important to consume other sources of calcium to avoid deficiency of calcium and vitamin D. Some other foods that are high in calcium include Kale, Bok choy, broccoli, chia seeds, sesame seeds, and canned sardines.

Constipation

Constipation is a common symptom in IBD patients just as it is in the general population. It is important to determine if constipation is a result of a complication of IBD such as intestinal obstruction, vs simple constipation. If there is intestinal obstruction, there will also be significant abdominal pain, vomiting, and abdominal distension. Rectal inflammation, also called proctitis, can lead to difficulty with passage of stools giving a sensation of constipation, often associated with a sense of urgency (have to run when you have to go) and incomplete evacuation (still feel like there is more even after a bowel movement). There may also be bright red bleeding or mucus with bowel movements.

If there is no evidence of intestinal obstruction or rectal inflammation, simple measures can be used to treat constipation.

One can feel constipated either due to infrequent bowel movements or due to having to strain for the passage of hard stools.

Hard stools are indicative of dehydration and imply that more water/liquids need to be consumed. In general, it is important to have 64 oz. of water per day. This requirement may be increased when the weather is hot, with dehydration due to heavy sports and sweating, or if there is profuse diarrhea. Caffeinated beverages such as coffee, tea, and soda do not count as suitable liquids for hydration and can actually cause dehydration because of their diuretic effect, resulting in increased urination and water loss.

A high fiber diet helps. 25–30 g of fiber a day is the optimal amount of fiber for the average person. It is important to consume sufficient water with fiber. The fiber absorbs water and becomes soft, expands and stretches the colon to stimulate adequate colonic contractions. This allows easy stool passage. It would help to print a chart that lists the fiber content of different foods and place it somewhere visible so that one may calculate how much fiber one is obtaining per day. The following website offers a comprehensive list of foods and their fiber content.

https://www.dietaryguidelines.gov/resources/2020-2025-dietary-guidelines-online-materials/food-sources-select-nutrients/food-0

If dietary intake is insufficient, over the counter fiber supplements can be used as well. Soluble fiber such as psyllium is best and should be taken in powder form, dissolved in a large glass of liquid. Fiber gummies are acceptable if sufficient liquid is consumed with them, but can sometimes disintegrate and adhere to the esophagus causing symptoms of esophageal pain.

"P" fruits, i.e., fruits beginning with the letter "P" contain high amount of soluble and insoluble fiber and can help to relieve constipation. Examples include peaches, plums, pears, pineapple, papaya, and prunes. Prunes are particularly useful because they also contain sorbitol, a fermentable sugar that can have a laxative effect.

If the above measures fail, there are medications that can be used to treat simple constipation including over the counter laxatives such as senna and MiraLAX, and stool softeners such as Colace.

If simple measures fail, it is important to bring this problem to the attention of your doctor so that they may evaluate further and come up with a treatment plan. For severe IBS-C constipation, there are prescription medications that can relieve constipation. Need for this is rare in IBD.

Diarrhea

Diarrhea is a common problem in IBD. It is important to treat the cause of the diarrhea before treating the diarrhea itself. If there is no inflammation and the IBD is in remission but there are still frequent loose stools, consider other causes such as irritable bowel, infections, or dietary intolerance.

Simple measures that can help symptomatically include a low fiber diet. Low fiber foods include refined starches like white breads and pasta, meats, fish, and chicken. Anti-diarrheals should not be used without first consulting with your doctor because their use may cause complications in colitis if there is active inflammation. Avoid caffeine and alcohol as they can increase diarrhea.

Pain Management

In General

Avoid NSAIDs such as aspirin, Ibuprofen (Advil), Naproxen (Aleve), as they can cause a flare of inflammation and bleeding. Tylenol, if taken according to recommended dosage is safe. If there is preexisting liver disease, Tylenol should be taken with care and only after checking with a physician.

Abdominal Pain

The primary focus should be to determine the cause of the pain and treat that. Inflammation of the intestine can cause pain. Once the inflammation resolves, the pain too resolves. Generally, pain medications are not recommended because they can mask a serious illness. In some rare cases, chronic abdominal pain due to complicated Crohn's can be managed with the use of antidepressants, making use of their neuromodulating properties.

Rectal Pain

It is important to see your doctor if you are having rectal pain. It can be caused by many things including hemorrhoids, fissures, fistulae, or pus pockets and will need specific treatment.

Emotional Support

There are numerous strategies that can be used to cope with IBD. For example, if diarrhea is a predominant symptom, knowing where restrooms are in places commonly visited would be useful. Carry extra underwear and wipes. The Crohn's and Colitis Foundation of America (CCFA) can provide a card which patients can use in order to have access to bathrooms in restaurants, etc.

If traveling for a long period of time, it is important to have enough medication on hand and develop a plan which includes establishing care with doctors in the area you are visiting.

The CCFA organizes support groups that can be very useful for new patients. Discussion with patients who are familiar with the disease can ease anxiety and allow for learning coping strategies from others. The local chapter of the organization also provides mentoring facilities and informational meetings. Developing a support group of friends and family that can help during stressful periods is important. Sometimes taking a family member with you to doctor's office appointment can ease anxiety and stress and provide someone else to remember instructions.

Mental Health

Living with any chronic condition can cause significant anxiety, stress, feelings of loneliness, and sometimes depression. Stress in turn can aggravate symptoms of IBD leading to a cycle of illness. It is therefore important to discuss this aspect of one's health with your physician and, if necessary, seek counseling with a psychologist or psychiatrist. Some medications used for the treatment of depression can alleviate gut pain and symptoms, due to their pharmacologic effects in the gut. Modulation of pain is an important aspect of these medications.

Regular exercise, yoga, and engaging in activities and hobbies that you like will also help ease anxiety and stress. There are generally no restrictions on exercise, but it is prudent to check with your doctor before engaging in any serious exercise program. If you have a stoma, check with your surgeon before engaging in abdominal exercises.

Education

Educating oneself about IBD is one of the keys to a successful partnership and a good therapeutic relationship with your doctor. It is however important to be selective in your research because there is misinformation online that can significantly affect one's perception of IBD and its treatments. Good options include the Crohn's and Colitis Foundation of Ameerica (CCFA), Medline plus, and information produced by IBD clinics and centers. Other options include books such as this. Attending workshops and seminars are also good ways to network with other patients and care givers and educate yourself. See Appendix.

Living with an Ileostomy/Colostomy

Living with a stoma can be very difficult and life changing. The adjustment should begin prior to surgery if possible. There are many resources available including the CCFA and stoma nurses who often work with your surgeon. They can answer many commonly asked questions and help relieve anxiety.

It is common to feel sad and ashamed, but it is important to realize that you are not alone. Consider seeing a mental health counselor or joining a support group for people with stomas.

Plan ahead when you go out to eat or drink because you may have to empty the pouch.

You should not need special clothes because, most times, the pouch will lay flat against your body. There should be no restrictions on activity either, but heavy lifting may harm the stoma. Always check with your doctor before embarking on any strenuous exercise program. Many people with stomas are runners, lift weights, ski, swim and play most sports. It is a good idea to empty your pouch before you start exercising.

Intimacy is probably the greatest concern for patients with stomas. It is important to have good communication with your partner and discuss your and their concerns openly. Again, a counselor may be useful. The stoma nurse may be able to give you a special wrap to cover the stoma in order to help you feel more secure.

The Ileal Pouch Anal Anastomosis (IPAA) or "J Pouch"

In most instances, quality of life with a pouch improves due to fewer bowel movements and urgency compared with active UC in an intact colon. Most patients should be aware that they will have at least 6 bowel movements a day after the IPAA. If there are significantly more bowel movements or other symptoms associated with it, such as pain or urgency, contact your doctor as it may be an indication of inflammation, called pouchitis. Pouchitis may require specific treatments, sometimes via a suppository/enema, sometimes with tablets and sometimes with immunomodulators and biologics. Rarely, the pouch may need to be revised surgically or removed altogether and converted into an ileostomy.

Fertility is often reduced in women after IPAA surgery. Conversations regarding childbearing and fertility, if relevant, should take place prior to surgery. It is unclear what the exact cause of infertility is, but it is believed to be secondary to manipulation within the pelvis during the operation. However, IVF success rates appear to be similar in women after IPAA compared with women in the general population. In men there may be a low risk of impotence, which should also be discussed prior to surgery.

Most patients with IPAAs live productive and fulfilled lives.

Chapter 10
Fertility and Pregnancy with IBD

Many women are diagnosed with IBD during their childbearing years. This causes concerns and questions regarding fertility, pregnancy, the baby's health, and safety of medications. In fact, some women choose not to have babies due to unfounded concerns and misconceptions. It is very important to have this conversation early in the treatment process as it may affect which medications are used.

Fertility

Fertility refers to the ability to get pregnant and carry a healthy baby through delivery. There is no difference in fertility between women in the general population and women who have well-controlled IBD. However, there is some evidence that active inflammation in CD or UC may result in reduced fertility and pregnancy rates. In addition, there is a reduction in fertility after some pelvic surgeries such as the IPAA as outlined in the previous chapter. It is unclear what the exact causes are but maybe related to scarring around the uterus and gynecological organs.

One concern that patients have is whether any of the medications for IBD can interfere with fertility. As far as we know, none of the medications interfere with fertility in women. However, sulfasalazine (Azulfidine) can cause low and abnormal sperm counts in men, leading to the inability to impregnate a woman. This is reversible. It takes about 3 months for sperm production to normalize after the medication is stopped. Therefore, it is best to avoid using this drug in any man who is trying to get his partner pregnant.

Methotrexate may cause mutations in sperm and therefore infertility and should be avoided in men who are trying to impregnate their partners.

R. Rajapakse, *Crohn's Disease and Ulcerative Colitis*, https://doi.org/10.1007/978-3-031-45407-3_10

Inheritance of IBD

There are over 200 genes identified in association with IBD, but none is linked to causation. This is likely due to the fact that IBD is believed to result from an inter-mingling of various factors such as genetics and external triggers. Having one of the IBD genes doesn't mean that one would develop IBD and not having the gene does not mean that one would never develop IBD. Genetic testing is therefore not routinely performed outside research facilities.

If there is one first degree relative with IBD (mother, father, brother, sister), the risk of getting IBD is about 10%. If there are two first degree family members with IBD, for example, both parents, the risk of having a child with IBD becomes closer to 30%. Most of this data is from Caucasian studies. IBD also appears to be most common in Caucasians especially Ashkenazi Jews and less common in Hispanics, Asians, and Africans.

Prior to Pregnancy

It is important for any woman with CD or UC who is contemplating getting pregnant to have a discussion with their physician. In general, the best time to get pregnant is when IBD is in remission. When IBD is in remission, outcomes of pregnancy are similar to those of the general population. If you are in a flare(meaning if the disease is active), your physician may advise delaying pregnancy until remission has been achieved because there is a slightly higher risk of spontaneous abortions, premature delivery, and small babies when the mother has active inflammation. It is also an important time to discuss birth control issues, nutritional issues, and genetic issues in addition to treatment. Smoking cessation and optimizing nutrition should be discussed. It is important to start prenatal vitamins and to address any nutritional deficiencies prior to pregnancy.

The timing of pregnancy will determine what the best treatment options are. No medication can be guaranteed 100% safe during pregnancy. We do know however that a flare of IBD is more deleterious to pregnancy than most of the medications in current use. In general, most medications that maintained remission before pregnancy can be continued, after discussion with your physician.

Medication Safety During Pregnancy

Aminosalicylates (5-ASAs)

These are of different chemical structure than aspirin and are generally safe. Please see above for consideration of sulfasalazine in males. If a woman is taking sulfasalazine, it is important to take adequate folic acid. Sulfasalazine can deplete the body of folate, and folate deficiency during pregnancy can cause neurological problems in the fetus/embryo.

Steroids

Steroids should not be used as maintenance treatment in IBD. Every attempt should be made to start an effective maintenance treatment and discontinue steroids prior to pregnancy. However, if this is not possible, or if a woman has a flare of IBD during pregnancy, steroids can be used safely. Steroids are old drugs and have been used safely for other conditions during pregnancy such as asthma. Although in animal studies they have been associated with birth defects, many years of experience in pregnant women with IBD and asthma have not revealed similar problems in humans. The lowest dose and shortest course should be used, if feasible.

6-Mercaptopurine (6-MP)/Azathioprine(AZA)

These drugs have been in use for IBD since the 1980s. If a patient is in remission on one of these drugs prior to becoming pregnant, they should be continued because they are considered safe during pregnancy. However, if a patient is on a combination of a biologic and 6-MP or AZA, an attempt should be made to discontinue one of them when they are planning pregnancy due to a possibly higher risk of infections in the baby when the mother receives dual therapy. Usually the 6-MP/AZA will be stopped and the biologic continues. Again, the risk of stopping one of the medications has to be weighed against the risk of a possible flare.

Methotrexate

This drug is a teratogen and can cause congenital malformations in the baby if the mother is exposed during pregnancy and is contraindicated in pregnancy. In general, it is best to avoid using this drug in women of childbearing age to avoid exposure in the event of an unplanned pregnancy. If a woman of childbearing age is prescribed this drug, adequate and effective contraception should be mandated. If a woman is planning to get pregnant and is already on methotrexate, the drug should be stopped at least 3 months prior to planned conception and an alternative medication is used for controlling of IBD.

Biologics

The anti-TNFs are the oldest of the biologics and have a lot of evidence of safety during pregnancy. There is some passage of infliximab across the placenta in the third trimester, but it does not appear to harm the baby, so most experts do not recommend holding the medication. Most of the data comes from safety registries. So far it appears that Entyvio and ustekinumab are safe too. It is important to discuss these medications with your physician if pregnancy is being planned. Ultimately risks of the drug must be weighed against carrying a pregnancy safely to term because we know that the biggest threat to a healthy pregnancy is active disease.

There is insufficient information about the safety of Xeljanz, Zeposia, and Skyrizi during pregnancy.

If a man is planning on impregnating his partner, all the medications except for sulfasalazine can be continued. Methotrexate may be continued with caution to ensure that the pregnant partner does not come into contact with it.

During Pregnancy

It is important to keep up with regular appointments with the gastroenterologist and obstetrician. If there are special circumstances, your doctor may want you to be followed by a high-risk Ob. It is important to continue all medications prescribed by your physician and have routine lab work to prevent flares. According to medical data, about one-third of patients in remission before getting pregnant will flare during pregnancy.

If there is a disease flare during pregnancy, the patient should be managed by a gastroenterologist who has experience caring for pregnant IBD patients. Options for management will be carefully considered and may include getting additional tests, changing medications, a course of steroids, or admission into the hospital.

Lab and stool tests may be ordered to check for electrolyte abnormalities, kidney or liver dysfunction, anemia, and evidence of inflammation. If required, an endoscopic procedure is safe in the second trimester but should be avoided, if possible, in the first and third trimesters. MRI does not produce radiation and can safely be performed without contrast, during pregnancy. Plain abdominal X-rays produce minimal radiation and can also be safely performed. Ultrasound is useful for evaluation of the gall bladder and liver, should that become necessary, and is also safe to perform during pregnancy.

Medications should be continued as outlined above, under the guidance of a physician. This is important so as to prevent a flare of disease.

Delivery

Most IBD patients can have an uneventful vaginal delivery. If there is significant perianal disease such as fistulas or abscesses, then it is best to avoid vaginal delivery. Vaginal tears or an episiotomy (a cut made by the physician to facilitate delivery) may not heal well and can worsen the perianal disease.

If there is an ileal pouch anal anastomosis (IPAA) or "J pouch," either Cesarian section or vaginal delivery can be performed safely depending on the obstetric needs of the patient.

The best mode of delivery for a pregnant IBD patient should be determined by collaboration between the gastroenterologist, the Ob/gyn, and the patient.

Breast Feeding and IBD Medications

Most medications used for treatment of IBD are safe during nursing and breast feeding.

Biologics (infliximab, adalimumab, certolizumab, vedolizumab, and ustekinumab) seem to have an acceptable safety profile for breastfeeding.

Targeted small molecules: JAK inhibitors (tofacitinib, Rinvoq, Zeposia), not enough data to make a recommendation regarding breast feeding safety.

5-ASAs: Acceptable safety. May occasionally cause diarrhea in the breast-fed infant.

Azathioprine/6-MP: Acceptable.

Steroids: Prednisone has an acceptable breastfeeding safety profile. It is best to delay breast feeding for 1–2 h after the dose.

Budesonide: Acceptable breastfeeding safety.

Antibiotics: Augmentin: Acceptable, Cipro: acceptable. Delay breastfeeding for 3–4 h after dose.

Methotrexate and Metronidazole (flagyl): Breast feeding is contraindicated while on these medications.

Vaccination of Infant

Live vaccines should be avoided in the infant for 12 months post-delivery if the mother received biologics during pregnancy, after discussion with pediatrician and gastroenterologist.

Chapter 11
Special Concerns in Pediatric and Elderly Patients with IBD

Pediatric IBD

Inflammatory bowel disease can present for the first time at any age, and it poses a unique set of problems in pediatric patients.

While UC tends to present more in adulthood, Crohn's tends to be the more frequent presentation in children. There is also an entity called Very Early-Onset IBD (VEO-IBD), when IBD is present in infants. Pediatric patients, babies, children, and teenagers have unique challenges and problems compared to adults.

Symptoms

In children, IBD manifests with similar complaints to adults. There may be abdominal pain, diarrhea, bloody diarrhea, fevers, nausea, and vomiting. They may also have symptoms outside the intestines such as joint pains, skin rashes, eye pain and redness, mouth ulcers, and jaundice. Sometimes children simply have only a failure to grow according to milestones. This may be due to a poor appetite and inability to eat or due to an inability to absorb nutrients from chronic inflammation. If the IBD is not treated appropriately, and poor nutrition continues, chronic illness can result in a final height lower than expected according to growth charts and heights of family members. Sometimes there is also delayed puberty. It is therefore important to evaluate further any child who is not growing adequately or who has a delay in puberty even without overt symptoms suggestive of IBD. There are, of course, numerous causes of growth failure in children, IBD being only one of them.

R. Rajapakse, *Crohn's Disease and Ulcerative Colitis*, https://doi.org/10.1007/978-3-031-45407-3_11

Diagnosis

Similar to adults, a detailed history will be taken by the pediatrician. Family history is also important. The physician will order lab tests to check for inflammatory markers, hemoglobin, liver tests, and kidney tests. Stool samples will check for inflammation and any evidence of infections. Endoscopic procedures will be ordered in order to visualize the intestinal lining and to take tissue samples (biopsies). CT scans or MRIs may be ordered to visualize the entire abdomen and the small bowel. Capsule endoscopy will aid in visualizing the small intestine. The pathologist will look at samples and determine if there is any evidence of chronic inflammation to suggest IBD.

Treatment

Just as in adults, there are two phases of treatment: induction of remission and maintenance of remission. Some of the drugs that are used to bring the disease into remission may be used to maintain remission and some are not. For example, steroids are used to induce remission particularly in UC but should never be used as a maintenance treatment because of their potentially serious side effects.

In UC, the goal of treatment is to heal the lining of the mucosa and to get rid of symptoms, thus allowing normal growth and development. Similar goals are present in Crohn's, but complete healing of the lining may be more challenging. The ultimate goal is to halt inflammation and prevent complications such as growth failure, intestinal narrowing, fistulas, abscesses, etc., as has been outlined in other parts of this book. It is very important to persevere and use the available medications judiciously and, at the same time, know when it is not working and switch to a different agent. Therefore, being cared for by a pediatrician who specializes in IBD is important.

As in adults, induction treatment includes steroids and anti-TNFs. A key difference between management of pediatric IBD and adults is that nutrition has been shown to make a significant difference to inflammation in pediatric patients.

Treatment should be tailored to the patient as well as the location and severity of diseases. So, for example, inflammation of the ileum alone is treated differently from inflammation of the colon alone. Some forms of mesalamine may be used for mild inflammation. For more severe disease, a steroid may be needed to induce remission. Steroids should never be used for long-term treatment due to their potential side effects which in pediatric patients includes growth failure.

Maintenance of remission may be achieved with mesalamine in patients with colonic inflammation alone but usually requires an immunomodulator or biologic agent. As in adults, immunomodulators used include 6-MP/azathioprine or methotrexate. If there is concomitant arthritis, methotrexate may be a better option as it can treat both arthritis and IBD. Anti-TNFs (Infliximab and Adalimumab) have been extensively used in pediatric and adult populations and are a very good option as well. None of the other biologics have been approved by the FDA for use in children and adolescents. The choice of treatment will be determined by the physician based on the extent of the disease, severity, other coexisting illnesses, and patient preference.

Response to treatment will be monitored by improvement in symptoms (such as abdominal pain and diarrhea), imaging such as CT scan and MRIs, colonoscopy, lab work, and stool tests.

Levels of medication in the blood can also be measured in order to ensure an optimal response. If there is a lack of response, efforts should be made to optimize dosing or switch to another agent.

Nutritional Modalities

These have been studied extensively in the pediatric population and found to be effective when compared to standard therapies, especially in CD.

Ulcerative colitis appears to be much less amenable to nutritional interventions in children in terms of reducing inflammation, but elimination diets can sometimes result in improvement in symptoms.

It is important to consult with a gastroenterologist and nutritionist when considering dietary therapy for inflammatory bowel disease to ensure that all the necessary nutritional components are ingested daily to maintain adequate growth and health.

Exclusive Enteral Nutrition (EEN)

This involves replacing all regular food with a liquid formula that contains all the necessary nutrients. These formulas contain the calories, carbohydrates, proteins, and fats that are needed for growth and health. Their use is more popular in Europe than in the USA. In Europe, it is considered the first line of treatment for pediatric patients with Crohn's disease. EEN is not as effective in adults as it is in children.

EEN helps to reduce inflammation and therefore reduces symptoms such as pain and diarrhea. It also helps with weight maintenance or weight gain. Overall, it can improve the quality of life.

EEN is used usually in the short term to induce remission, and then regular foods are gradually reintroduced. In this situation, it may be used for 4–12 weeks. It works best when it is used correctly, i.e., avoiding other foods and fluids while on EEN. It can be drunk like a regular drink but if this is not possible, it can also be given via a tube that is passed from the nose into the stomach.

It can be difficult to get used to using EEN as a sole source of nutrition. Always check with the dietician and prescribing gastroenterologist but some tips to make it tolerable and filling include the following:

- Drinking it cold and sipping slowly
- Blending with ice to make a frappe

- Drinking it warm
- Space out or alternate different flavors
- Spread the drinks throughout the day to prevent hunger

Once the prescribed period for induction is completed, the dietician will assist in helping to re-introduce foods by interspersing regular food with the EEN. The dietitian will determine how fast or slowly this should be done and will also suggest a meal plan that will provide the necessary nutrients.

EEN is very safe and effective when used correctly. The major drawback is tolerability and the need to avoid regular food. The support of family and friends helps with this aspect of the treatment, and they should be included in discussions. Many other diets have been tried and promoted in the media for adults and children with IBD, but have not shown actual healing.

Specific Carbohydrate Diet (SCD)

In this diet, certain carbohydrates are eliminated from the diet, and some aren't. It was initially developed for patients with celiac disease but received more notoriety in IBD. This diet is based on the theory that some undigested carbohydrates are fermented by bad bacteria in the gut causing more inflammation and symptoms. Most positive responses have been via patient testimonials but medical evidence for efficacy is lacking. In this diet, sugar, grains, starchy tubers such as potatoes, sweet potatoes, and all dairy are not allowed.

Although studies to date have not shown significant efficacy with treatment of Crohn's disease and ulcerative colitis in terms of reducing inflammation in the intestine, this diet does seem to help with symptoms. This is not surprising because many symptoms such as bloating, and diarrhea can be produced by bacterial fermentation of non-digested carbohydrates.

The Crohn's Disease Exclusion Diet (CDED)

This diet involves the elimination of processed foods and is usually combined with Partial Enteral Nutrition (PEN). It is particularly useful for patients who cannot tolerate EEN. There is some data that this diet can reduce inflammation and produce corticosteroid free remission in children with Crohn's disease.

Surgical Treatment

Surgery is reserved for children who have intractable disease that has failed medical treatment, or who developed complications.

In Crohn's disease, this can include the development of abscesses, fistulas, perforation, bleeding, or obstruction due to narrowing of the intestines. Often, when there is an element of scar tissue, medical therapy is no longer effective, and the patient will require surgery.

In the case of ulcerative colitis, again surgery is indicated if there is intractable disease in spite of medical treatment or if there is a complication. Complications that can occur in ulcerative colitis include toxic megacolon (where the colon becomes very large and close to perforation), bleeding, or perforation (the colon develops a hole in it). In children who have significant disease, it is important to involve a surgeon in management at an early stage, even if surgery is not imminent. This allows the child to build a relationship with the surgeon and also to familiarize themselves with the possibility of surgery and the potential surgical options.

It is important to remember that surgery is not curative for Crohn's disease and long-term therapy with medications will still be required after the surgery. On the other hand, ulcerative colitis is cured with surgery and usually does not require any further medical therapy unless there is remaining colonic tissue left behind, or if there is inflammation of the anal pouch or a change in diagnosis.

Very Early-Onset IBD (VEO-IBD)

This is defined as inflammatory bowel disease that occurs before the age of 6. Infantile IBD is a distinct subset of VEO-IBD that develops in children less than 2 years old. About 10% of pediatric IBD patients present before the age of 6 years. IBD is uncommon in children, but IBD in this age group seems to be increasing in incidence over the past few years.

It appears that genetics plays a larger role in patients who present at a young age and the IBD may be more resistant to treatment.

It is very important to have a multidisciplinary approach when treating patients with VEO-IBD, including a gastroenterologist, immunologist, geneticist, hematologist, nutritionist, and surgeon depending on the clinical presentation and presence or absence of manifestations outside the gut. Referral to a center with expertise is usually necessary.

In general, it is important to be certain of the diagnosis and to rule out other causes, such as infections and celiac disease in the first instance.

If a genetic defect is identified, targeted gene therapy may be used. Sometimes a stem-cell transplant may be necessary depending on the genetic problem that has been identified. Immunomodulators can be used as well. Biologic therapy does not seem to work well in very early-onset IBD compared to the general pediatric population.

Pediatric to Adult Transition

As with all chronic diseases, it is important that pediatric patients with IBD have a smooth and seamless transition from the pediatric gastroenterologist to an adult gastroenterologist. The question always arises as to what age this should take place. The American Academy of Pediatrics defines pediatric care from birth through age 21. However, every child is different, and some children may be ready to see an adult gastroenterologist even sooner. It is important that the child has the independence and skills to take on self-care, such as making appointments with the physician, understanding medications and their purposes, and taking medications independently. It is also important for the pediatrician to provide comprehensive medical records as well as a personalized transition note to the adult gastroenterologist in order to make it easier for the patient. Some practices have transition clinics during which a child can see their pediatrician as well as an adult gastroenterologist every couple of months and gradually transition entirely to the adult clinic. This should be discussed with the pediatrician and gastroenterologist early on, to reduce stress for the child and family.

Elderly Onset IBD

Although the peak age of onset of inflammatory bowel disease is between the ages of 30 and 40, there appears to be a second peak between the ages of 60 and 70 years. About 10–15% of cases are diagnosed after the age of 65. As people live longer, the prevalence of inflammatory bowel disease also appears to be rising in the elderly.

The definition of elderly onset IBD varies depending on the definition of older age, but it is generally accepted that IBD that occurs after the age of 60 is defined as elderly onset IBD.

Elderly Onset Ulcerative Colitis

Elderly onset ulcerative colitis appears to be more common on the left side, and less extensive than in younger patients. It also tends to be less severe. Surprisingly elderly patients tend to present more with constipation and straining rather than with bloody diarrhea.

Elderly Onset Crohn's Disease

Early-onset Crohn's disease tends to occur more in the colon than in the small bowel and again appears to be less extensive. It also tends to be less aggressive, which implies that the disease tends to remain in the initial location without too much spread. There is more inflammation and less narrowing or fistula formation compared to CD in adults.

In addition, manifestations outside the gut are less common in the elderly.

Treatment of Elderly Onset IBD

The same therapeutic modalities that are used in adult IBD are also used in the elderly. However, there are several factors that need to be considered in the treatment of elderly onset IBD. Elderly patients are more likely to have other illnesses such as heart disease, lung disease, diabetes, arthritis, and kidney problems which may impact treatment of IBD. Sometimes, the diagnosis of inflammatory bowel disease in elderly patients can also be challenging because of other conditions, such as ischemic colitis, which can mimic IBD. In ischemic colitis, blood supply to the colon is reduced, especially in patients with heart disease and problems with blood vessel, resulting in thickening and inflammation of the colon. This may be precipitated by dehydration. In addition, elderly patients have reduced immune function and therefore immunomodulators and biologics need to be used with caution.

The risk of surgery in elderly patients is higher than in the regular adult population due to the increased incidence of heart and lung disease.

Colorectal cancer risk increases with age and with duration of inflammatory bowel disease but there does not appear to be any increased risk of colon cancer in the elderly onset IBD patients compared to regular adult onset. However, there is an increased risk of lymphomas in elderly onset IBD compared to regular IBD even without the use of immunomodulators and biologics.

Chapter 12
Routine Health Maintenance, Vaccination, and Screening

In general, it is important for anyone, with or without IBD, to focus on maintaining health and avoiding disease by eating a healthy diet, exercising regularly, and getting the recommended screening procedures and interventions at the appropriate time. This is especially important in patients with IBD because the disease itself, as well as some of the medications that are used for treatment, can predispose them to other illnesses. For example, long-term Crohn's of the small bowel can predispose to poor appetite and reduced intake as well as decreased absorption of calcium and vitamin D, resulting in bone loss. Many medications that are used to treat IBD can also cause other problems, see Table 12.1.

Most often, screening and routine health maintenance lies in the field of primary care physicians. However, in IBD, gastroenterologists will often initiate these screenings. It is important for patients with IBD to be aware of the important screening measures they should undergo, and bring them to the attention of their doctors, if they haven't been done.

Screening

All patients should undergo routine screening as recommended by their primary care physician. In IBD patients, particular attention needs to be paid to screening for colon cancer, cervical cancer, and skin cancers, particularly in patients on immunologic and biologic therapies (Table 12.2).

Table 12.1 Complications that can be associated with IBD medications

Medication	Problems
Steroids (prednisone, hydrocortisone, solumedrol)	Bone loss, osteopenia, weight gain, cataracts, diabetes
6-MP, azathioprine	Skin cancer, lymphoma, low blood counts, infections, cervical cancer
Biologics: Remicade, Humira, Cimzia, Entyvio, Stelara, Skyrizi, biosimilars	Infections, cancer, skin rashes, allergies
Small molecules: Xeljanz, Rinvoq	Infections, cancer, thrombosis, cholesterol abnormalities

Table 12.2 Current preventive health maintenance recommendations from the American college of Gastroenterology

After 8 years of pancolitis	Colon cancer screening with colonoscopy
Women on immunosuppressants	Consider pap smears every 1–2 years
All patients but especially on biologics and immunomodulators	Routine skin checks especially after age 50
All patients, especially with steroid use	Bone density periodically
All patients	Consider screening for depression and anxiety

Screening for Colon Cancer

Colon cancer occurs more commonly in patients with UC and in Crohn's of the colon, compared to the general population. The risk increases with the duration of disease, the extent of disease, and the severity of disease. Therefore, patients with colitis affecting the whole colon have a higher risk of colon cancer than patients with only left-sided colitis. In addition, patients with rectal inflammation alone don't seem to have an increased risk of colon cancer compared to the general population. It appears that chronic inflammation is the predominant driving factor for cancer and therefore the aim of treatment should be to achieve healing of the lining whenever possible. The risk of colon cancer is increased if there are other factors at play such as a family history of colon cancer, history of smoking, sedentary lifestyle, and frequent consumption of red meat.

It is therefore important to have regular colonoscopies as indicated below:

Colonoscopy every 1–3 years starting 8–10 years after the symptom onset of colitis.

During the colonoscopy, multiple biopsies are taken randomly throughout the colon. These samples are inspected under the microscope by the pathologist looking for dysplasia. Dysplasia is an abnormality that occurs in the cells before there is cancer. If dysplasia is found it is graded into low- or high-grade dysplasia. Depending on the finding, the gastroenterologist may recommend a colectomy or more frequent and intensive colonoscopies. Sometimes the gastroenterologist will spray a blue dye during the colonoscopy. The blue dye can enhance any abnormal area of the colon allowing easier detection. The usual agent used is methylene blue. It makes the stool and urine blue for about 24 h after the procedure. The endoscopist may also use blue light called Narrow Band Imaging (NBI) to inspect the colon. When surveilling for dysplasia and cancer, it is important to try and achieve remission prior to doing the colonoscopy.

Patients with primary sclerosing cholangitis and IBD require more intensive surveillance because they are at higher risk of colon cancer. They are also at risk for bile duct cancers and therefore require blood tests and imaging on a regular basis.

Patients with Crohn's of the small bowel may be at risk for cancer of the small bowel but there is no routine surveillance recommendation.

Pap Smear for Cervical Cancer

Cervical cancer and dysplasia are largely related to the human papilloma virus (HPV), and therefore vaccination at the age-appropriate times is the best way to prevent cervical cancer. There are studies that have shown a higher incidence of cervical cancer in patients on immunomodulators such as 6-MP and azathioprine and therefore it is recommended that these patients undergo more frequent pap smears, i.e., every year rather than every 3 years as is recommended for the general population. All adult female IBD patients should establish care with a gynecologist.

Bone Health

Bone loss and osteoporosis are well-known problems in post-menopausal women. Osteoporosis is a condition where the bone becomes weaker and therefore becomes increasingly amenable to trauma and fractures. Many factors contribute to bone health, but an adequate intake of calcium and vitamin D is especially important. Therefore, if the diet is poor or there is an inability to absorb, as may occur in bad Crohn's of the small intestine and after surgical resection of the small bowel, bone loss, and osteoporosis can result. The biggest cause of bone loss however is steroid use in IBD.

Therefore, it is recommended that a baseline bone density scan is obtained on any patient with risk factors, and on a periodic basis thereafter. If bone loss is detected, it should be treated, and the scan can be repeated every 2 years.

Improving bone health requires the following:

- Smoking cessation
- Weight bearing exercises
- Avoiding excessive alcohol intake
- Quitting cigarette smoking

- Calcium and vitamin D supplementation (age 19–50, calcium 1000 mg/day, women 51–70 1200 mg/day)
- Avoiding or judicious use of steroids
- Treating the primary disorder effectively if possible

Screening for Skin Cancer

Most light skinned people, especially those who have spent a prolonged time in the sun during their youth, are at risk for skin cancer and should get routinely examined by a dermatologist. IBD patients are particularly at risk for non-melanoma skin cancers. This includes squamous cell cancer and basal cell cancer. It is believed that this risk is mainly due to the use of immunomodulators and biologic agents. It is very important that patients on these treatments take measures to decrease sun exposure with the use of protective clothing and high index UV protection. In addition, these patients should undergo yearly full body skin checks with a dermatologist.

Screening for Depression and Anxiety

Depression and anxiety are more common in IBD patients due to the chronic nature of the disease, and because it can have a significant impact on quality of life. It is important to recognize this and discuss it with the health care provider. Depression can become a barrier to medical treatment of IBD resulting in worsening disease. Some practices provide access to psychologists, but if they don't, patients should consider seeking counseling with a licensed provider. Many patients feel that there is a stigma attached to it. It is important to realize that depression is extremely common in any chronic illness and becomes almost a part of the whole disease process which must be addressed in order to regain full health.

Cigarette Smoking

Cigarette smoking is associated with significantly higher risk of Crohn's flares and complications such as strictures, abscesses, and fistulas. Therefore, in addition to the general and cardiovascular benefits of smoking cessation, it becomes especially important in Crohn's disease. There are many different pharmaceutical options and non-pharmaceutical options available. Some people benefit from hypnotherapy, exercise, and acupuncture, while others need medications. Some of these medications can have side effects which should be taken into consideration prior to use. All of this should be discussed with your health care providers, both gastroenterologists and primary care physicians.

Vaccinations

Table 12.3 lists the vaccinations recommended by the American College of Gastroenterology for patients with IBD:

Medications used for the treatment of IBD such as steroids, biologics, and immunomodulators, can increase the risk of infection. Therefore, it is particularly important for these patients to be vaccinated. 6-MP/AZA and Some of the newer medications used for the treatment of IBD (small molecules) cause an increased risk of shingles. Therefore, these patients are particularly advised to get the new inactivated shingles vaccine.

Influenza is one of the most preventable illnesses by vaccination for which there has been abundant data. Prior to the advent of this vaccine, influenza season was accompanied by a significant number of hospitalizations and death. Influenza still accounts for a significant number of hospitalizations during the season which extends through winter and spring. There are two vaccines available: a live one administered in the nose, and an inactivated one administered by injection. Patients on immunosuppression should receive the inactivated vaccine.

Pneumococcal vaccine: It is currently recommended that all patients over the age of 65 receive the pneumococcal vaccine. All patients with IBD over the age of 19, on immunosuppressants are at a higher risk for pneumococcal pneumonia and should therefore be vaccinated with the pneumococcal vaccine. There are two pneumococcal vaccines that cover the whole range of potential types of pneumococcal pneumonia and IBD patients should receive both.

Shingles vaccine: Chicken pox is caused by the virus called varicella zoster. Once someone has had chicken pox, which may at times be subclinical, the virus can reactivate causing very painful skin blisters that may occasionally become complicated by neuralgias and other complications. Combination therapy with an anti-TNF and an immunomodulator as well as some of the new medications (small molecules) approved for treatment of IBD can produce an increased risk of shingles. Therefore, patients who require these drugs should be vaccinated against shingles.

The current shingles vaccines available in the US is inactivated. The previously used live vaccine is no longer available in the US. Shingrix, the inactivated vaccine, is recommended for IBD patients on immunomodulators/biologics. The vaccine is given as 2 injections 2–6 months apart and may cause pain at the injection site. This vaccine appears to be 90% effective in preventing shingles in IBD patients.

Table 12.3 Vaccinations recommended for IBD patients

All adult patients	Annual influenza vaccination: inactivated if patient is on biologics/immunomodulators
All adults patients	Consider pneumococcal vaccine
All adult patients>50	Shingles vaccine
Adolescents	Meningococcal vaccine
All patients	Age-appropriate vaccinations

Other Vaccinations

All patients are routinely screened for hepatitis exposure prior to initiation of immunosuppressive treatments because latent viral infections can reactivate.

Hepatitis A is transmitted by the fecal-oral route and can cause a GI illness, with liver abnormalities, that is usually self-limited. All patients should be vaccinated according to CDC guidelines. This vaccine can provide protection for 10–20 years depending on the immune system of the patient.

Hepatitis B is transmitted through body fluids and also during childbirth from the mother, especially in Asian countries.

50% of patients with latent hepatitis B can experience reactivation especially if on immunosuppressives. If latent infection with hepatitis B is noted, it can be treated at the same time as immunosuppressives/biologics are administered in order to prevent reactivation. If there is no evidence of exposure or immunity, patients should be vaccinated prior to receiving a biologic.

Hepatitis C is also believed to be transmitted by body fluids. If there is evidence of infection, it should be treated prior to initiating immunosuppression. There is currently no vaccine for Hepatitis C.

Most IBD gastroenterologists will refer patients with liver disorders or hepatitis to a hepatologist (a liver specialist) in order to manage that part of the illness.

Nutrition

Patients with IBD may suffer from particular nutritional deficiencies.

Calcium and Vitamin D: this is discussed under bone loss.

Vitamin B12: This is a vitamin that is important for maintaining adequate hemoglobin and for nerve function. It is stored in the liver for many years. It is absorbed in the last part of the small intestine, the terminal ileum. Crohn's patients with inflammation or resection of the ileum may develop a deficiency of this vitamin. It is only found in animal products and fortified cereals, so strict vegans may also become deficient. Initially vitamin B12 deficiency does not produce any symptoms and may only be picked up with blood tests. Severe deficiency can cause anemia and neurological problems such as pins and needles, numbness, and problems with balance and coordination. If there is a deficiency of vitamin B12, it should be supplemented with injections or the nasal formulation because the oral formulations may not be adequately absorbed.

Iron: Iron is important for the formation of hemoglobin and to prevent anemia. It is found in many foods and absorbed in the small intestine. Again, patients with Crohn's of the small intestine, surgical resection or bleeding can become iron deficient. Sometimes the bleeding is not overt and may only be microscopic. Inflammation itself, even without bleeding, can lead to iron deficiency.

In the early stages, iron deficiency will not produce any symptoms but when significant anemia develops, it can cause fatigue and shortness of breath with exertion.

Iron can be replaced orally or by intravenous infusion. Unfortunately, oral iron can have GI side effects such as abdominal cramping and a change in bowel habit. Slow-release formulations are better tolerated. There are intravenous formulations that are administered usually by a hematologist. These are well tolerated. Treatment of the underlying inflammation, in combination with a well-balanced diet, will also result in normalization of hemoglobin.

Other considerations are as follows:

Use of Marijuana

Cannabis sativa, known as marijuana is well known for its psychogenic effects. However, there are also cannabinoid receptors in the GI tract, and some IBD patients find it useful for modulating pain and cramping. There is no data to show that it improves inflammation in IBD patients. In addition, chronic use can result in nausea and vomiting and "hyperemesis syndrome" causing even more problems in patients with IBD.

Other Interventions for Health Maintenance

Aside from a healthy diet as outlined elsewhere, modified to a particular patient's needs, exercise is also important for good health. Chronic illness can be a significant source of stress for patients, and this can be addressed in a variety of ways. As mentioned above, seeking care from a mental health professional can be helpful. Sometimes medication may be required. Nonpharmacological strategies are also useful. These include acupuncture and mind body therapies such as meditation. These therapies can be used in conjunction with conventional treatment but should not replace it.

Chapter 13
Extra-Intestinal Manifestations of IBD: Manifestations Outside the Gut

Although IBD primarily affects the gut, it can also cause problems outside the GI tract. These problems may precede, occur at the same time, or occur after the diagnosis of IBD. Often the symptoms go unnoticed by the patient and the doctor until the diagnosis of IBD is made. Common sites affected include the skin, the eyes, joints, liver, and blood.

Up to 40% of patients with IBD will have problems outside the GI tract. They tend to occur more in women than in men.

Skin Manifestations

The most common skin manifestations of IBD are erythema nodosum and pyoderma gangrenosum. Both of these conditions can occur with other diseases as well. There are other rare skin conditions that can occur with IBD.

Erythema Nodosum

Erythema nodosum can occur in many diseases other than CD. It is associated with tuberculosis, bacterial infections, malignancies (lymphoma), some medications, and pregnancy. It occurs in about 15% of IBD patients, more commonly in Crohn's than in UC. It produces tender, well-defined red lumps most commonly on the shins. It usually tends to occur during a flare of Crohn's. Diagnosis is made by history and physical examination. Treatment has to focus on the underlying condition but in severe cases, steroids may be required to calm it down. EN can go into remission for extended periods, especially when the underlying IBD is under control.

© The Author(s), under exclusive license to Springer Nature Switzerland AG 2023
R. Rajapakse, *Crohn's Disease and Ulcerative Colitis*,
https://doi.org/10.1007/978-3-031-45407-3_13

Pyoderma Gangrenosum (PG)

This is the second most common skin manifestation of IBD, but it is rare, occurring in about 1–2% of patients. It tends to be more common in women.

It produces painful skin ulcers anywhere in the body, but more commonly in areas that have been traumatized, for example, in scars and at the site of stomas. It is diagnosed clinically. The ulcers are tender, can be very small to very large, with pus in the base, and are painful. Occasionally, a biopsy is needed. Treatment can be difficult and includes steroids and cyclosporine either as a cream or orally. The anti-TNFs also appear to be effective in healing PG, and it can go into remission for an extended period of time.

Psoriasis

Patients with psoriasis have a higher risk of developing IBD compared to the general population, especially UC. Sometimes there is an associated psoriatic arthritis. Psoriasis, like IBD, is an immune-mediated disorder. Psoriasis produces red scaly patches that tend to occur on the elbows and knees but can occur anywhere. Fortunately, there are several medications currently available that can be used for the dual purpose of treating IBD and psoriasis, with good results.

Anti-TNFs have been used to treat psoriasis but can sometimes cause psoriasis in patients. If this occurs, management depends on severity. If the psoriasis is mild, it can be treated while the anti-TNF is continued. However, if it is severe, the anti-TNF may have to be discontinued for an alternative treatment.

Medication Side Effects

Many medications can cause an allergic-type reactions producing red bumps. The medication may have to be discontinued, and the allergy treated with benadryl or sometimes with steroids.

Mouth

Mouth problems are more common in CD and in Males. Mouth ulcers, gum lesions, and tongue lesions can occur. Treatment includes mouth washes, steroids, and treatment of the underlying IBD.

Eye Problems

Eye manifestations are produced by inflammation of various parts of the eye. Inflammation can produce uveitis (inflammation of the colored part of the eye), scleritis, and episcleritis (inflammation of the white of the eye). Depending on the site of inflammation, it can produce a localized redness in one part of the white of the eye or a complete red eye. There may or may not be blurred vision or pain in the eye. In any case, redness and any eye symptoms should always be taken seriously because delaying treatment can lead to vision loss. It is important to see an ophthalmologist for diagnosis and treatment as soon as possible. Treatment involves treatment of the underlying IBD and use of anti-inflammatory drops in the affected eye.

Arthritis

Joint problems are common in IBD. Arthritis can affect the "central" joints meaning the spine, or "peripheral" joints such as knees, hips, hands, and feet. It can also affect small (fingers, feet) or large joints (hips, shoulders). It occurs more frequently in women and is often attributed to regular "osteo" arthritis which people get with advancing age. Often arthritis follows the course of inflammation in the bowel so when there is abdominal pain and diarrhea, joint pains can occur at the same time. Joint pain can be accompanied by stiffness and limited range of movement.

Diagnosis is made by a rheumatologist using clinical history, physical examination, lab tests, and X-rays.

Treatment again is that of the underlying IBD as well as arthritis. There are many medications that are useful for treating both arthritis and IBD and should be selected based on their dual efficacy. Steroids and NSAIDs should be avoided if possible. Physical therapy is often useful as well.

Liver Manifestations

Primary Sclerosing Cholangitis (PSC)

This is a condition that affects the bile ducts in the liver causing inflammation and scar tissue formation. Eventually the inflammation can cause narrowing of the ducts leading to obstruction of bile flow and jaundice. It does not produce symptoms in the early stages and may be suspected only due to abnormal liver tests noted on routine blood testing. MRI of the liver may demonstrate it, but definitive diagnosis often requires a liver biopsy.

PSC can predispose to a higher risk of bile duct cancer and colon cancer. Therefore, patients with both PSC and IBD have to be surveilled more closely with colonoscopies and imaging.

There is no effective treatment for PSC. Severe disease may be treated with a liver transplant.

Other Manifestations

IBD can also produce problems in the lungs and the kidneys. Lung problems include certain types of noninfectious pneumonias and inflammation.

The kidneys may also be affected by inflammation, and kidney stones can occur in both CD and UC. The urologist may want a stone to identify its composition. Depending on the type of stone, dietary modifications or specific solutions may be prescribed.

Bone Loss

Prolonged use of steroids or significant disease activity (as has been described elsewhere) can lead to osteoporosis: bone loss. This can cause increased risk of fractures. Periodic bone scans, called Dexa scans, can be performed to assess bone density. If there is a concern, calcium and vitamin supplements can be used. In more severe cases, specific medications may be prescribed.

Blood Clots

There is an increased risk of blood clots in IBD. This is especially so in women with IBD who are taking oral contraceptive pills. The lowest dose of hormone pill should be used. Precautions should be taken on long flights, etc., such as stretching legs and walking around. Hospitalized patients should have preventive measures such as compression stockings to prevent clots.

Medication Side Effects

All medications used for the treatment of IBD can have potential side effects outside the GI tract. These include but are not limited to anemia, infections, skin rashes, kidney and liver problems. Therefore, whenever there is a new diagnosis, it is important to review all medications to ensure that they are not causing the problem.

Chapter 14
Last Thoughts

Keep a Log

Because Crohn's and colitis are chronic diseases, so it is a good idea to keep a concise log from the time of your IBD diagnosis. It does not have to be very detailed, or long, because it is important that it should not be too hard for someone to review. It can be an excel spread sheet, an exercise book with tabs that you can update as time goes on, or a folder into which you can insert pages. The log should contain the most important information:

- Date of diagnosis, and how long you had symptoms before the diagnosis, how was diagnosis made, e.g., colonoscopy.
- Extent of inflammation if known, i.e., entire colon, colon and ileum, only small bowel, etc. Ask your doctor.
- Any complications? E.g., Abscesses, fistulas, perforation, etc.
- Number of hospitalizations, dates, and which hospitals.
- Medications tried for IBD and why they were stopped. E.g., side effects (what side effects) or "didn't work."
- Number, dates, and type of surgeries and why it was done, e.g., small bowel resection for a narrowing and obstruction or because "medication didn't work."
- Dates of colonoscopies (month and year), at least the most recent ones. Try and keep a copy of the reports.
- Most recent labs. (Try and keep a copy). Labs from many years ago are usually not useful.
- Other diseases/illnesses. E.g., Diabetes, heart failure, etc.
- An updated list of all medications you are taking,
- List of vaccinations,
- List of most recent health maintenance, e.g., mammogram, colonoscopy, skin checks, etc.

© The Author(s), under exclusive license to Springer Nature Switzerland AG 2023
R. Rajapakse, *Crohn's Disease and Ulcerative Colitis*, https://doi.org/10.1007/978-3-031-45407-3_14

This log will be an "aide memoire" for you and will be invaluable to any physician who takes over your care. This is especially useful if you change doctors.

Financial Concerns

IBD often affects people during their peak earning years. This can pose a significant financial strain on the patient and their family. Non-working patients may not have access to insurance, and this affects their ability to pay for treatments.

Most of the newer treatments for IBD, especially the biologics, are very expensive with few "generic" or non-branded alternatives.

It is very important to bring up any financial concerns with your doctor so that you can work together to find the best treatment alternatives.

Antibiotics are relatively cheap and can be used for some specific conditions such as anal fistulas or inflammation of a J pouch. There are generic alternatives to many antibiotics.

Mesalamine also is a generic product. All mesalamine products are not the same. Even though the active drug is the same, they are formulated differently to be released in different parts of the gut and to have different properties. Most insurance companies will have a couple of mesalamine products at least on their formulary. Sulfasalazine, the oldest 5-ASA product is also inexpensive but can be used to treat only colonic inflammation and does not work for inflammation of the small intestine.

Immunomodulator medications like 6-MP and AZA are covered by most insurances and are relatively inexpensive even without insurance.

Biologic therapies are prohibitively expensive without insurance. Most insurers do cover biologic treatments but may only cover a bio similar, i.e., a biologic therapy similar to the brand name. Some drug companies have patient assistance programs: ask your doctor. Some insurance companies require you to have failed certain biologics before another can be prescribed. This can lead to delays in receiving the most appropriate medication.

It is vital that these financial issues are brought to the attention of the prescribing physician so that less expensive alternatives can be prescribed. Sometimes a physician's office can appeal to the insurance company to pay for medication after a one-to-one discussion with a physician from the insurance company. This does not always work.

Changing Doctors/Moving out of State or Country

If you keep a log of your illness, it will be invaluable in your transition to a new doctor.

Your doctor or the CCFA can provide recommendations regarding IBD specialists in your new location. It is preferable to register with an IBD specialist rather than a generalist, especially if you have had a complicated course. It is important that medication is not interrupted. Interruptions of biologics can cause your body to start rejecting it. If this happens, it can produce an allergic reaction and may not be effective anymore. Medication interruptions can also produce flares of disease activity leading to further stress for the patient.

Request that your current doctor sends pertinent records to your new doctor including dosage and timing of infusion therapies in order to ensure a seamless transition.

Travel-Related Concerns

Travel is always a source of anxiety for patients with IBD for many reasons. The best guarantee of a stress-free experience is to be in remission before travel. Anticipate how long you will be traveling for and make sure to take sufficient medications with you. If traveling for an extended period of time, be prepared to make the acquaintance of a physician at your destination. Your doctor may be willing to discuss your care with a physician abroad if necessary.

If you are on biologic infusions, discuss timing of the infusions in relation to travel with your doctor so that there is no extended interruption.

If you are taking biologic injections, and it is due while you are away, make sure to take a supply with you and ensure that it is stored appropriately in order to avoid spoilage.

If you are taking immunomodulators/biologics, pay special attention to food hygiene, especially when traveling to areas of the world with a high incidence of traveler's diarrhea. It is prudent to only drink bottled water and to use the same for teeth brushing. Avoid eating salads and pre-cut fruits unless you prepare it yourself with appropriate precautions. Take a supply of Pepto-Bismol and Imodium with you and discuss travel with your physician prior to travel. Also keep some medication for constipation in your travel medication kit, such as Dulcolax or MiraLAX sachets. If you have diarrhea, ask your physician if taking Imodium is appropriate while on vacation. In this era of COVID and respiratory infections, it is prudent to wear a mask in any particularly crowded environment.

Biologics/immunomodulators can predispose to non-melanoma skin cancers. Remember sun protection, especially while on vacation. Physical sun protection, such as hats and long-sleeved garments, is best but if this is not possible, use sufficient SPF and remember to re-apply regularly, especially if swimming.

Many patients with diarrhea are afraid of driving any distance because of the need for bathrooms. The CCFA has a card that identifies a person as having IBD and can be used to request use of a bathroom anywhere. In addition, it would be useful to know where there are bathrooms on frequently used routes.

Work/School-Related Concerns

Many patients who are working or in school will experience significant hardship when they are in a flare of IBD. This may be due to being unwell with abdominal pain, nausea, etc. or due to the need to make frequent trips to the bathroom. It is useful to have an honest discussion with your supervisor regarding your needs even if they are intermittent. Your doctor can often provide a note for work or school to allow absences for illness, medication infusions, and frequent bathroom breaks.

Appendix

Recommended Resources

https://www.crohnscolitisfoundation.org/
https://www.dietaryguidelines.gov/sites/default/files/2020-12/Dietary_Guidelines_for_Americans_2020-2025.pdf
https://www.healthline.com/health/soluble-vs-insoluble-fiber#recommendations
https://www.webmd.com/ibd-crohns-disease/crohns-disease/low-residue-diet-foods
https://www.drugs.com/cg/lactose-controlled-diet.html
https://www.niddk.nih.gov/health-information/digestive-diseases/lactose-intolerance
https://www.healthline.com/nutrition/low-fodmap-diet#steps

© The Editor(s) (if applicable) and The Author(s), under exclusive license to
Springer Nature Switzerland AG 2023
R. Rajapakse, *Crohn's Disease and Ulcerative Colitis*,
https://doi.org/10.1007/978-3-031-45407-3

Index

A

Abdominal pain, 62
Abscesses, 54
Active inflammation, 43
Acupuncture, 85
Allergic reactions, 31
American college of Gastroenterology, 80
Aminosalicylates (5-ASA), 67
Anal sex, 12
Anemia, 14
Anti Saccharomyces antibody (ASCA), 22
Antibiotics, 28, 35, 69
Antibodies, 31
Anti-depressant medications, 18
Anti-neutrophil antibody (ANCA), 22
Anti-tumor necrosis factor (anti-TNFs), 30, 34, 72, 88
Anxiety, 82
Aphthous ulcers, 8
Arthritis, 89
Augmentin, 69
Azathioprine (AZA), 32, 33, 56, 67, 69, 72

B

Bacterial fermentation of non-digested carbohydrates, 74
Benadryl, 88
Bifidobacterium, 38
Bile, 4
Bile duct cancers, 81
Biliary system, 1
Biliary tract, 5
Biologic agents, 31, 56

Biologic therapy, 54, 75, 92
Biologics, 28–31, 64, 68, 69, 83, 93
Biosimilars, 30
Birth control issues, 66
Blood clots in IBD, 90
Blood markers for inflammation, 27
Blood tests, 21, 26
BMI calculator online, 44
Bone health, 81, 82
Bone loss, 81, 90
Breast feeding, 69
Budesonide, 32, 69

C

Calcium, 84
    blood vessels, 47
    decreased absorption, 47
    dietary sources, 47
    hormones, 47
    muscles and nerve function, 47
    steroids, 47
    strong bones, 47
    supplementation, 47
Calcium deficiency, 47
Cancer, 14
Cancer risk, 31
Cannabidiol (CBD), 39
Cannabinoid receptors, 85
Cannabinoids, 39
Cannabis, 39
Cannabis sativa, 85
Capsule endoscopy, 25, 26
Carbohydrates, 74

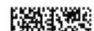